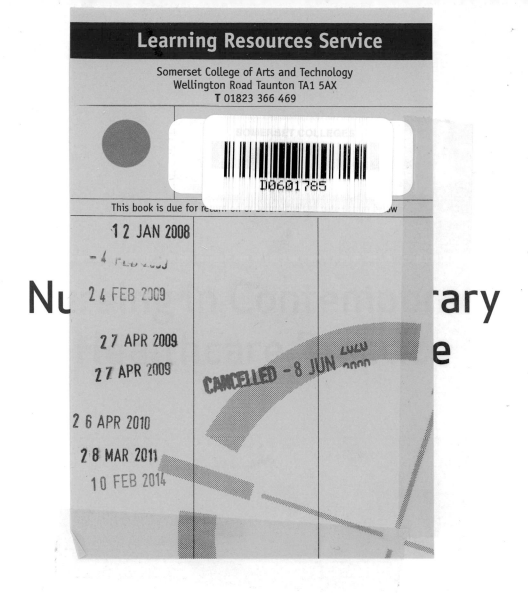

Series Editor: Shirley Bach

Transforming Nursing Practice – titles in the series

Law, Ethics and Professional Issues in Nursing   ISBN 978 1 84445 160 9
Nursing and Working with Other People   ISBN 978 1 84445 161 6

To order, contact our distributor: BEBC Distribution, Albion Close, Parkstone, Poole, BH12 3LL. Telephone: 0845 230 9000, email: **learningmatters@bebc.co.uk**. You can also find more information on each of these titles and our other learning resources at **www.learningmatters.co.uk**

Nursing in Contemporary Healthcare Practice

Graham R. Williamson, Tim Jenkinson
and Tracey Proctor-Childs

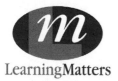
LearningMatters

First published in 2008 by Learning Matters Ltd

British Library Cataloguing in Publication Data
A CIP record for this book is available from the British Library

ISBN: 978 1 84445 159 3

The right of Graham R. Williamson, Tim Jenkinson and Tracey Proctor-Childs to be identified as the authors of this Work has been asserted by them in accordance with the Copyright, Designs and Patents Act 1988.

Cover and text design by Code 5 Design Associates
Project Management by Diana Chambers
Typeset by Kelly Gray
Printed and bound in Great Britain by TJ International Ltd, Padstow, Cornwall

Learning Matters Ltd
33 Southernhay East
Exeter EX1 1NX
Tel: 01392 215560
E-mail: info@learningmatters.co.uk
www.learningmatters.co.uk

Contents

Abbreviations

A & E	Accident and Emergency (Department)
BMA	British Medical Association
BME	Black and Minority Ethnic
BMJ	*British Medical Journal*
BRII	Bristol Royal Infirmary Inquiry
CE	clinical effectiveness
CEA	cost-effectiveness analysis
CFP	Common Foundation Programme
CHAI	Commission for Healthcare Audit and Inspection
CHI	Commission for Health Improvement
CNO	Chief Nursing Officer
DH	Department of Health
EBP	evidence-based practice
EOC	Essence of Care
EPP	Expert Patient Programme
EPT	Expert Patient Trainer
ESC	essential skills cluster
EU	European Union
GNC	General Nursing Council
GP	General Practitioner
HAI	hospital-acquired infection
HCP	healthcare professional
HE	higher education
HEFC	Higher Education Funding Council
HEI	higher education institution
ICN	International Council of Nurses
KSF	Knowledge and Skills Framework
LTC	long-term condition
LTCA	Long Term Conditions Alliance
NCAA	National Clinical Assessment Authority
NHI	National Health Insurance
NHS	National Health Service
NHSE	National Health Service Executive

NICE	National Institute for Health and Clinical Excellence
NMC	Nursing and Midwifery Council
NPFN	National Pension Fund for Nurses
NPSA	National Patient Safety Agency
NSF	National Service Framework
OSCE	objective structured clinical examination
PA	Patients Association
PBC	practice-based commissioning
PCT	Primary Care Trust
PFI	private finance initiative
QAA	Quality Assurance Agency
RBNA	Royal British Nurses' Association
RCN	Royal College of Nursing
RCT	randomised controlled trial
SHA	Strategic Health Authority
SSRN	Society for State Registration of Nurses
UKCC	United Kingdom Central Council for Nursing, Midwifery and Health Visiting
VAD	Voluntary Aid Detachment
WDC	workforce development confederations

Foreword

It is not often that you find a book that brings different aspects of the diverse discipline of nursing together in one text. For example, in preparation for registration as qualified nurses, students can follow one of four branches to learn how to care for adults, children, persons with mental health problems or with learning difficulties. Following registration, there are approximately 60 subspecialties of nursing that concentrate on very different areas such as cardiology, community nursing, forensic nursing, diabetes, and so on. By tracing the early beginnings of the formation of the National Health Service, Graham R. Williamson, Tim Jenkinson and Tracey Proctor-Childs outline the history of modern-day nursing and its many branches and specialities. They skilfully lay before us the foundation of ideas that have shaped the contemporary healthcare practice we know today. The approach the authors have taken, to take a look back in time, helps us understand where we are going in the future and is therefore an excellent compass for student nurses and future qualified practitioners.

The book explores, in depth, nursing policy-making and politics, and will be essential reading for nursing students to grasp the intricacies of the influences that shape our profession. Having inside knowledge can equip nursing students to be informed and effective advocates for their patients as well as future lobbyists for their profession.

There are essential themes in the book that closely relate to the current climate of healthcare practice. The authors explore the caring culture that pervades our work and the impact current issues of gender and multiculturalism have on today's practice. The crucial role that evidence-based practice plays in underpinning current practice and ensuring that the quality agenda are achieved are also highly relevant themes. These are dealt with in the text by providing very current material, in what are known to be changing and dynamic topics. The concluding chapters provide pertinent insights to the student experience and patient perspective, and will help to prepare students for their journeys into healthcare practice.

In each chapter the relevant NMC Standards of Proficiency are stated and will be a feature of the Transforming Nursing Practice series. This ensures that nursing students will see exactly how the information in the book relates to achieving their competencies and be ready to practise in the contemporary world of nursing we know today.

Shirley Bach
Series Editor

Introduction

This book examines issues related to the context in which care is delivered; that is, how factors relating to the organisation of the National Health Service (NHS) have had an impact on how nurses go about their work. The book is organised into chapters, each with a separate theme, but the chapters' themes are related.

In Chapter 1, 'The establishment of the National Health Service', we will examine how healthcare was organised before the NHS was established; its history and policy from its establishment in 1948 to 1997; NHS structures, acute and community care, and the mixed economy of welfare. Chapter 2, 'Contemporary issues in healthcare policy', continues our analysis of the NHS by focusing the discussion on more contemporary issues, following the election of a Labour government in 1997.

In Chapter 3, 'Nursing, policy making and politics', we will look at areas where politics, policy making and nursing practice intersect. We will begin by looking at how the law relating to nursing registration has changed over time. Next, we will look at some influences on political parties' health policies and their impact on government and Parliament. Then we will examine the media's influence on the health policy agenda, in the form of press and television reporting. Finally, we will look at the role of trade unions and the Royal College of Nursing (RCN) and their influence on health policy, and the role of the RCN as the nurses' professional body.

Chapter 4, 'The caring culture and tradition in nursing', examines some issues concerning concepts of caring. We will begin with a brief mention of the impact of two key figures in the history of nursing, Florence Nightingale and Mary Seacole. They lived in a very different society from our own, and we will link their work to more contemporary ideas about what caring is and how it is affected by gender issues and multiculturalism in today's health service.

In Chapter 5, 'Evidence-based practice', we consider the recent development of EBP in healthcare decision making and how it can enhance clinical effectiveness by allowing us to make judgements about which treatments and procedures work, rather than relying on custom and practice alone. This chapter introduces some basic EBP concepts appropriate to Common Foundation Programme (CFP) level students.

Chapter 6, 'Quality in healthcare', examines various considerations ranging from the costs of healthcare to the recent political developments and media representation of quality issues, arguing that 'quality' remains elusive and is something that can differ from person to person. Even so, many different tools, benchmarks,

1

targets and milestones have been set up by government in order to raise standards and improve the quality of service provision in the NHS.

Chapter 7 is named 'The student experience' and examines various issues concerning being a student nurse in a higher education setting involving clinical placements. It includes material on study skills and time management, reflection and portfolio writing, and on attending university, working in placement areas, undertaking assessments of practice and the importance of relationships with mentors. It will also look at professionalism and becoming a registered practitioner, registering with the Nursing and Midwifery Council, and the CFP and the branches of nursing.

In Chapter 8, 'The patient perspective', we provide you with some important insights into the type of skills you will need to develop in order to become a partner in care with the patients you meet. At the centre of your role as a student of nursing is the practice of good communications skills, through which you can demonstrate respect and consideration for the patients in your care. Listening to their concerns and responding in a helpful, supportive and positive manner will help some people to develop the confidence they need to make decisions about their own conditions and treatment.

Finally, Chapter 9, 'Conclusions and future directions', reflects on material covered in preceding chapters and highlights developments that are on the horizon at the time of writing, and that are likely to have an impact on nurses and their careers as we progress through the early twenty-first century. Key areas of future change are briefly summarised, and there are links to suggested websites for further reading.

NMC *Standards of Proficiency*

The Nursing and Midwifery Council (NMC) has established standards of proficiency to be met by applicants to different parts of the register, and these are the standards it considers necessary for safe and effective practice. This book is aimed at first-year student nurses in all branches in the Common Foundation Programme (CFP), and is structured so that it will help you to understand and meet the standards required for entry into the branch programme; that is, gain progression from the CFP to your chosen branch. The standards are presented at the beginning of each chapter so that you can easily see which standards the chapter addresses. Most have CFP standards, and occasionally branch standards are listed. They are mandatory, in accordance with legislation, and are taken from the 'Standards of education to achieve the NMC standards of proficiency, Standard 7 – First-level nurses' in *Standards of Proficiency for Pre-registration Nursing Education* (NMC, 2004).

Activities

Throughout the book you will find activities in the text that will help you to make sense of, and learn about, the material being presented by the authors. This book contains a mix of theoretical material at an appropriate level for the first-year CFP student and practical applications, meaning that the activities will enable you to see the relevance of the text to everyday practice situations. Some activities ask you to reflect on aspects of practice, or your experience of it, or the people or situations you encounter. Reflection is an essential skill in nursing, and it helps you to understand the world around you and often to identify how things might be improved or carried out more effectively in the future. All the activities require you to take a break from reading the text, think through the issues presented and carry out some independent study, possibly using the internet. Where appropriate, there are sample answers presented at the end of each chapter, and these will help you to understand more fully your own reflections and independent study. Remember, academic study will always require independent work: attending lectures will never be enough to be successful on your programme, and these activities will help to deepen your knowledge and understanding of the issues under scrutiny and give you practice at working on your own.

Chapter 1

The establishment of the National Health Service

Chapter aims

After reading this chapter, you will able to:

* understand why the NHS was established in 1948;
* summarise its development until 1997;
* understand the benefits of provision for clients in the independent sector;
* appreciate the relationship between management and clinicians in your current placement area.

Introduction

In this chapter we will examine how healthcare was organised before the NHS was established, its history and policy from its establishment in 1948 to 1997, NHS structures, acute and community care, and the mixed economy of welfare. In the next chapter, we continue our analysis of the NHS by focusing the discussion on more contemporary issues, following the election of a Labour government in 1997.

Pre-NHS healthcare in Britain

The organised healthcare of the NHS was not achieved as a revolutionary idea, although the establishment of the NHS in the post-war period was a 'watershed' or 'tipping point' in that central government intervened on a large scale effectively to nationalise the healthcare sector after World War II (WWII). Before this, healthcare needs were met in a variety of ways, and in Britain service provision had grown since the mid-nineteenth century, as charity, voluntary and church organisations established facilities for the poor and needy, with local authorities providing a range of services. Central government passed health-related legislation, particularly for public health regarding clean water, factory conditions and the control of infectious diseases. A system of health insurance was established in 1911 to provide a basic minimum when workers were unwell, and there was also some healthcare as part of poor law provision (Webster, 2002). In the period up to the beginning of WWII, local government and voluntary provision expanded but provided nowhere near comprehensive coverage: for example, nearly half the population qualified for the post-1911 National Health Insurance (NHI), but this only gave them access to general practitioner services not hospital care, and excluded the unemployed, dependants and children (Baggott, 2004).

It is by no means certain that a universal national system would have come about without WWII, but the war made it imperative that British healthcare was better organised as massive military and civilian casualties were anticipated; the voluntary sector still played an important part until it did. In the interwar period (1918–39) there were 1,000 independent, self-governing charity or voluntary hospitals, and 3,000 local government facilities, without any system of co-ordination or control. They differed in that, traditionally, the charity hospitals relied on donations for their funding, charged the rich for treatment and cared for the poor for free. However, it was difficult for the poor to get admission to them. By 1938, these hospitals were often short of funds, and were charging patients for treatment, caring for about one third of sick people at this time. Local government controlled other hospital facilities, often targeted at specific illnesses such as infectious disease, tuberculosis and mental problems, with some provision for maternity care. In addition, local authorities had responsibility for the Poor Law hospitals and the workhouses in which the less deserving poor were forced to live until these establishments were abolished in 1929. Early attempts following the Royal Commission on the Poor Laws in 1909 to establish the principle of free healthcare for the poor by right were dismissed as too radical (Baggott, 2004).

Many of the country's poor lived in squalid housing conditions, and, although the Victorians had made great advances in public health by providing clean water and sewerage in cities and towns following the 1848 Public Health Act, there were still great inequalities in the health of the rich and the poor, reflecting the great inequalities in income. Working-class women had the worst health status. They were not covered by the post-1911 NHI system, they usually lived on incomes below accepted poverty levels even when their husbands were working, and they were often required to deny themselves healthcare and decent food in order to maintain a healthy breadwinner husband and for the sake of their children (Webster, 2002).

Activity 1.1

Imagine that you live in London in 1900. Your husband is ill and requires costly treatment; as he is the only breadwinner his health needs get priority: how must it feel to prioritise his treatment above that of your children or yourself?

• Write down the sorts of emotions that you might experience.

There is a brief outline answer at the end of the chapter.

Activity 1.2

The term 'public health' has been used in the preceding discussion.

• What is your understanding of the term 'public health'?
  o Write down your own definition, and then look up the term in textbooks and on the internet. Write a paragraph summarising the information you have found. How does your definition compare to those you have found?

A sample answer is provided at the end of the chapter.

The birth of the National Health Service

It is difficult for generations born after WWII in the United Kingdom (UK) to appreciate the impact that this major historical event had on British society. The country's infrastructure was badly damaged by bombing, and its people emerged from the war years victorious but battered. As part of the process of rebuilding society, the incoming post-war Labour government introduced the reforms first formulated by William Beveridge, a Liberal politician who later became a peer. A high degree of consensus emerged around the proposals for government to intervene in social welfare on a scale never before seen in Britain. The Beveridge Report (Beveridge, 1942) was thus established to provide services and assistance *From the Cradle to the Grave*, with a range of measures against the *Five Giants of Want, Disease, Ignorance, Squalor and Idleness*, by means of:

- services paid for largely out of general taxation;
- services that are free at the point of delivery;
- access determined by need alone.

The report demanded the introduction of family allowances to provide against poverty in families where the head of the household was working, the introduction of comprehensive health and education services, and that the government maintain full employment so that citizens were able to work and pay taxes to support the new welfare expenditure. A whole range of legislation was introduced immediately after the war:

- Education Act (Butler Act, 1944);
- Family Allowances Act (1945);
- National Health Service Act (1946);
- National Insurance Act (1946);
- Children Act (1948);
- National Assistance Act (1948).

It was in this context of post-war reconstruction that the NHS was born, although there had long been calls for the reorganisation of health services in this country, which were disorganised and ineffective in delivering the required standard of care for anything like a majority of citizens (Klein, 2006). After 1948, all in the population were guaranteed equality of access to healthcare, with clinical need alone determining treatment rather than the ability to pay. General principles applied to Scotland and Northern Ireland as well as to England and Wales, although the details, structures created and dates of legislation were slightly different throughout the UK.

The intention was to ensure that healthcare was delivered to all in a fair and efficient manner (Klein, 2006). Family practitioner services, including doctors (General Practitioners, GPs), dentists, pharmacists and opticians, and other community services such as nursing and midwifery, became part of the same organisation, providing care and also acting as a gateway for referrals to hospital consultants who would see patients requiring more specialised care, as well as to nursing and midwifery services in hospital. The service as a whole was overseen by the Department of Health (DH).

Although these services were initially all provided free of charge, it soon became apparent that government had underestimated the true costs of establishing them, and of salaries and wages. It was initially assumed that a large expansion of services in the early years would lead to a reduction in illness as the NHS cured all the illnesses in society; indeed, no one connected with the establishment of the NHS in the years before its inception really seems to have questioned the costs involved, assuming that they would be somehow acceptable (Klein, 2006).

In 1949 prescription charges were introduced and in 1951 charges were extended to dentistry and spectacles, prompting the Health Minister Aneurin Bevan to resign in protest (Klein, 2006). A principle was therefore established early on in the life of the NHS, still extremely relevant to this day, which is that demand for services will always be greater than the money available to supply them; that is, a service funded from taxation alone cannot meet all of the health needs of everybody in the country, not if government is required to spend tax revenues on other services such as education, social services and defence. Thus there will always be some element of rationing in public service health provision.

Nursing at the time was almost exclusively the preserve of women, and the culture of the time was that women were subordinate to men in all things, therefore doctors were the powerful decision makers in all spheres, a fact reflected in their much greater pay and by the generous financial settlement that the post-war government offered them to secure their support for the new NHS. In the post-war period, the status of nurses began to change and a more professional system of education and training was established, but, even so, this quotation from Rivett (1998) illustrates how women in nursing were seen within healthcare settings:

> No woman should take up the profession of nursing unless she is prepared for hard work, constant subordination of her will, and for continual self denial . . . She must be trustworthy, conscientious and faithful in the smallest detail of duty. She must be observant and possess a real power of noting all details about her patient. She must be promptly obedient and respect hospital etiquette . . . A nurse's manner to her patient should be dignified, friendly and gentle, but no terms of endearment should be used. She should surround herself with mystery for her patient and never discuss her own private affairs.
>
> (Probationer's notes, St George's Hospital, London, 1946 – a Probationer was a nurse in training)

Activity 1.3

In order to begin to understand how the role of nurses might have changed since 1946, work through the following exercises.

*   Although you may have limited experience of healthcare so far, think about the quotation from the St George's Hospital Probationer's notes.
    *   How has the image of women in society changed since 1946?
    *   How are nurses perceived in healthcare these days?
    *   What other qualities, if any, might a nurse need in today's healthcare settings?

A brief outline of what you might think about is at the end of the chapter.

The development of the National Health Service

From its early idealistically inspired beginnings, the NHS grew rapidly in the 1950s into a huge administrative machine, with strong control attempted from the central Ministry of Health and the minister responsible to Parliament for spending throughout the system. At the time it was considered that this centralised organisational structure would produce a more rational, advanced system, with high standards of care available to all, and a high degree of cost efficiency (Baggott, 2004). However, as time moved on this early optimism was shown to be unfounded.

The system was administratively split between hospital, GP and local authority services, and this distinction caused problems with its management. Funding was also an issue as budgets rapidly expanded. Doctors established their power base in the management of services as well as in clinical care, and the 1950s saw the creation of a consensus among the general public, politicians, the press and academic writers in health and social policy that publicly funded welfare services, including the NHS, were effective and appropriate. New hospital building programmes to replace outdated facilities were undertaken, new hospitals called 'district generals' began to be established in towns and cities, and the Salmon Report recommendations (Ministry of Health and Scottish Home and Health Departments, 1966) established a management and career structure for nurses.

Clinical care in the NHS was split between GPs (who remained as independent contractors), hospital and local authority services, meaning that resources were frequently used wastefully and the system as a whole was unco-ordinated. In 1973, the system was reorganised as a result of legislation, and area health authorities under district health authorities overseen by regional boards came to manage the services provided throughout the country for hospital services (secondary care), with family practitioner committees overseeing GPs, dentists and opticians (primary care), and local authority social services as a third strand in the structure (Wall and Owen, 2002).

Generally speaking, the period from the 1950s to the 1970s saw the 'welfare consensus' continue, with most people in Parliament and the country broadly in favour of taxation paying for improving public services. Influential academic authors such as Titmuss (1976) and Marshall (Marshall and Bottomore, 1992) captured the mood of the times by arguing that society had a duty to intervene to redistribute income through taxation, and that welfare services such as health were a major means by which social justice and social cohesion could be established and maintained: as everyone pays taxes and can access services, everyone has a stake in society, or so the argument went. At this time, the view was that citizens were automatically entitled to services and that by providing them society was demonstrating and expressing *higher values* (Bulmer et al., 1989) such as social justice; the welfare state was seen as a means by which income could be redistributed from rich to poor, as richer people paid a greater part of their income in taxes than did poorer people. Marshall (Marshall and Bottomore, 1992), for example, believed that the important things about politics and society were that there should be a *general enrichment* of the lives of citizens in the population, and that this could be achieved through welfare state spending. Needs, rights and citizenship thus became central ideas in these collectivist policies of the post-war era.

Thatcherite reform post-1979

However, this welfare state consensus began to erode as the 1970s wore on, and a Conservative government elected in 1979 took a radically different perspective that culminated in further NHS reorganisation in the 1980s and 1990s. Key influential academic authors at this time such as Hayek (1960) and Freidman and Freidman

(1980) argued that government spending on welfare had gone too far, taking away people's personal incentives to work, save and look after their own health. Thus, it was argued, a *dependency culture* had been created among the poor that undermined the *free market*, which, from this perspective, was inherently superior at organising production and distribution, and a *welfare bureaucracy* had been established that was unresponsive to the real needs of people because it operated only for its own benefits (Marsland, 1996). After 1979, Mrs Thatcher's government set about a radical restructuring of welfare services with the intention of fostering a new sense of self-reliance rather than welfare dependency, and a new emphasis on the needs of service users (consumers) rather than those of the professionals who deliver such services (Klein, 2006).

It had become clear that, as the NHS had budgets that were limited by the size of taxation, the service simply could not provide for every eventuality for every citizen in the country. Advances in medical technology and treatments, an increasingly older population and economic difficulties had put paid to the period of growth and consensus that had seen the NHS expand since 1948.

Key ideas for the NHS post-1979 were:

- competition among service providers;
- the introduction of general management;
- NHS Trusts;
- the purchaser/provider split;
- GP fund holding;
- the relocation of services away from the acute hospital sector;
- consumerism.

In 1983, the result of an NHS Management Inquiry, known as the Griffiths Report (Griffiths, 1983), was published. Its Chairman was Roy Griffiths, also Chairman of the supermarket chain Sainsbury's and a major supporter of the Conservative Party. The main elements of the report stated that:

- the NHS was suffering from institutional stagnation and it was impossible to effect change;
- health authorities were swamped with directives without being given direction;
- *consensus management decision-making* led to long delays in the management process.

The report famously concluded that:

> *if Florence Nightingale were carrying her lamp through the corridors of the NHS today she would almost certainly be searching for the people in charge.*
> (Griffiths, 1983, p17)

Three other factors were identified:

- **lack of managerial dynamism**: no driving force accepted direct, personal responsibility for planning, implementing and monitoring, and a more thrusting and committed style of management was required;

- **status quo orientation**: the NHS lacked real clinical or economic evaluation of its performance as a catalyst for change;
- **producer orientation**: it was questionable whether the NHS was meeting the needs of the patient and the community, and could prove that it was doing so.

The Griffiths recommendations were implemented almost completely, and general management was introduced into the NHS. General managers did not have a clinical focus – they were introduced with a remit for managing:

- finances and budgets;
- performance measurement;
- clinicians and others in the NHS.

This last area has been highly contentious, causing conflict in many settings between clinicians, particularly doctors, who previously had their power unchallenged in all spheres of the NHS (Klein, 2006).

Activity 1.4

In order to begin to understand relationships between key people and their roles in your organisation, work through the following exercises.

- In your current placement, identify the management structures. You might do this by looking at phone directories and the organisation's intranet and by talking to colleagues.
  - Who is the general manager?
    - What is his or her title?
    - What are the key roles and responsibilities?
    - To whom does he or she report?
  - Who is the lead clinician?
    - What is his or her title?
    - What are the key roles and responsibilities?
    - To whom does he or she report?
  - Who is the senior nurse?
    - What is his or her title?
    - What are the key roles and responsibilities?
    - To whom does he or she report?
- List the occasions on which you can identify them interacting over the course of two weeks.

As the answers will depend on your personal observation, there are no outline notes at the end of the chapter.

Activity 1.5

Having identified these key roles in your placement and the amount of inter-action that there is between them, reflect upon their interactions and answer the following questions.

- What were the interactions about?
- Did the people in these roles seem to be working as a team, or was one person 'in charge'?
- Who was 'in charge' and how do you know that they were?
- Were the interactions civil and courteous or not?
- Can you identify anything about the styles of interaction and communication that was good, bad or indifferent?
- How could the not so good aspects be developed?

There is a brief outline answer at the end of the chapter.

NHS and Community Care Act (1990) and a mixed economy of welfare

One key concern of the period after 1979 was the extent to which costs were rising, as the NHS at that time had responsibility for funding the care of older people, whose numbers were increasing as the population lived longer. A key piece of legislation was the NHS and Community Care Act (1990). This was an attempt to introduce radical reforms and to shift the setting for care away from the hospital sector by placing more emphasis on the community, individuals' relatives and friends, moving therefore towards 'community care' rather than in-hospital care and shifting the boundary for elderly care away from the statutory NHS, with its legal responsibility to pay for care, towards other sectors for which the state did not have the same legal duty for funding.

This had been a longstanding policy since the 1950s in mental health and learning disabilities care, as the large psychiatric hospitals were closed and services re-located. In mental healthcare, much critical work illustrated the destructive effects of removing ill and vulnerable people from their family and friends and local communities, and 'locking them away' in hospitals where the rules of life were very different. Goffman (1961), for example, produced a scathing attack on what he called *total institutions* such as hospitals, prisons, concentration camps, orphanages and barracks, categorising them as places where large numbers of similar people are cut off from the wider society for lengthy periods of time, and forced to lead a formally administered lifestyle.

These residential 'total institutions' and their inmates' separation from society meant that their self-concept (as parent, breadwinner or employee, for example) was completely altered. The individual's name, identity, personal belongings and so on were usually removed after admission and replaced by institutional codes and dress, thus explicitly stating that patients were no longer who they were; as Goffman (1961) puts it, they undergo *mortification of self* as total institutions change them. Immediately after admission they would undergo a series of humiliations and *profanations of self*, with the loss of basic rights such as privacy, dignity and self-determination eventually breaking down the individual's self-concept; inmates were punished if they did not co-operate. Goffman also believed that people were forced to adapt to the institution's rules, but most people do not maintain these adaptations permanently because they maintain the appearance of acceptance while actually protecting themselves. This might certainly have been the case for young prisoners or more lucid mental hospital patients. The more frail and vulnerable elderly person in a badly run long-stay unit may have had much less resistance. Staff were accustomed to receiving compliance, and took over from the individual all activities and responsibilities that they were used to carrying out for themselves in relation to their previous life. Individuals in total institutions did not plan their activities; they were planned for them, and this caused institutionalisation even if staff were well meaning.

It is for these reasons, as well as the financial one that the NHS could not continue to support increased activity in elderly care that the emphasis shifted away from institutional care and towards 'care in the community', with the continuation of the large-scale closure of NHS facilities for mental health, learning disabilities and elderly in-patient care, and a large expansion of such provision by the independent sector, voluntary bodies and charities.

Activity 1.6

In order to appreciate how your practice area welcomes and assesses patients and their care needs, and protects their rights and dignity, work through the following exercises.

- Think about how your current placement area admits patients.
  - Do staff introduce themselves?
  - Do they explain their roles?
  - Are they welcoming?
  - Is a full and holistic process of assessment undertaken?
  - Are patients treated as individuals?
  - Are patients expected to wear hospital clothes or can they keep their own?
  - How can patients complain about their services?
  - How are visiting times managed?
  - How are patients' privacy and dignity maintained?

As this activity is based on your own experience, there is no outline answer at the end of the chapter.

The 1990 NHS and Community Care Act aimed to improve the way in which the NHS and local authorities provided services, not just for mental health, but also for the elderly and those with learning difficulties, taking into account the Griffiths Report (1983) and the humanitarian criticisms of institutional care from Goffman

(1961) and others, implicitly if not explicitly. The Act required the development of partnerships of care between consumers, their representatives and with the voluntary and independent sectors, to provide a range of choices. The attempt was to foster a *mixed economy of welfare* with multiple service providers (meaning that the providers of care could be voluntary, charity, informal and NHS services) rather than services being delivered by the public sector alone; and also a shift away from institutional provision towards a service as close to clients' homes as possible. The 1990 Act gave a lead agency role to social services departments, who were to:

- stimulate service provision in the independent sector as opposed to providing the services themselves;
- publish community care plans on an annual basis following widespread local consultation;
- require care managers to assess need and produce flexible packages of care, and allocate key workers to cases.

In public relations terms, the language used was of breaking down barriers between institutions and the community, with the aim being to stimulate the empowerment of users and their carers (Means and Lart, 1994).

In addition, a government initiative called the Citizen's Charters began, indicating to consumers what could be expected of a range of state services. For health, the Patient's Charter (DH, 1992) set out the rights patients could expect from NHS services. These included the restated right to healthcare on the basis of need rather than the ability to pay, and service standards to be expected regardless of location, such as waiting list times and ambulance response times. Although criticised as being chosen only because they could be achieved, the Patient's Charter standards began to shift public thinking towards their entitlement to care and therefore away from the notion that they were only passive recipients of care. From 1993 comparative figures were published showing how well organisations had achieved these standards in relation to each other, and following this 'league tables' were introduced (Leathard, 2000). 'Named nursing' was introduced, whereby each patient was required to have an identified nurse to deliver and co-ordinate their care for the duration of their hospital stay or engagement with health services. This concept was similar in intention to primary nursing: to make clear lines of authority and responsibility for patient care in nursing by improving continuity. It was established in the belief that it would increase job satisfaction and contribute to *professionalising* nursing services (Steven, 1999), but was criticised as lacking substance and funding.

Activity 1.7

In order to begin to identify the provision for certain types of services and the boundaries that exist between them, work through the following exercises.

- In your local area, identify what kind of organisation – NHS, local authority and/or independent sector (maybe a charity or a private

> ### Activity 1.7 continued
>
> company) – provides the following services for clients, in order to discover what boundaries there are in service provision.
>
> - o Acute emergency care, for example following a heart attack.
> - o Long-term care of the elderly in nursing homes.
> - o Nursery provision for pre-school children with learning difficulties.
> - o Counselling and support of clients with alcohol and drug dependencies.
> - o Hospice services for the terminally ill.
>
> A brief outline of what you might find is at the end of the chapter.

The Health of the Nation

The Health of the Nation was a DH policy initiative White Paper that was intended to show the government's commitment to public health, to encourage improvements in service delivery and to foster attitudes towards healthy lifestyles in the general public. It was introduced by the Conservative government in 1992, and was a key English health policy until overhauled by the Labour government in 1997. It was an important innovation because it was the first explicit attempt by government to provide a strategic approach to improving the overall health of the population (Baggott, 2004).

Objectives were set in each of the five main areas of health and illness, with 27 targets set across these areas. Five main areas were:

- coronary heart disease and stroke;
- cancer;
- mental illness;
- HIV/AIDS and sexual health;
- accidents.

However, in research (DH, 1998c) conducted between 1997 and 1998, reviewers found that *The Health of the Nation*, although useful to focus attention on key areas for service improvement, had little real impact on service delivery or general health.

C H A P T E R   S U M M A R Y

- Although it is incorrect to say that, prior to 1948, all healthcare provision in the UK was dependent on the ability to pay, in the aftermath of WWII a comprehensive system was established, free at the point of delivery and dependent on clinical need. There was a split between GP services (primary care) and hospital care (secondary or acute care), with some local authority provision.

- This NHS was part of the welfare state, designed to look after UK citizens from the cradle to the grave.
- Although a subject of much support and consensus through its early years, by the late 1970s there was concern about rising budgets and lack of effective management and leadership, and a commitment to relocating services away from the hospital sector, including the involvement of charity and non-statutory provision in the independent sector (the *mixed economy of welfare*), and towards a more consumer-oriented service.
- Ideas such as consumerism, rights for patients and choice of services were established after 1979.
- These are important ideas for nurses to understand as they form the basis upon which contemporary NHS provision is founded.

Activities: brief outline answers

1.1 Husband's health needs (page 7)

The emotions reported will be very personal but are likely to be hopelessness, powerlessness, anger and fear, possibly leading eventually to resignation.

1.2 Public health (page 7)

Public health . . . *is primarily concerned with the efforts of the community to improve health, rather than the treatment of disease manifested in the individual* (Baggott, 2004, p336). It can encompass the promotion of health, the prevention of disease and the development of strategies to achieve these.

1.3 The changing image of women in society and in nursing (page 9)

- *How has the image of women in society changed since 1946?* Women in the UK in the twenty-first century have different images from those prevalent in 1946: particularly, their role in the workplace has changed so that they are legally entitled to equal treatment with men. Many more women work full-time and are often in positions of responsibility and authority in the workplace.
- *How are nurses perceived in healthcare these days?* Nursing in the twenty-first century has developed a new professional status, and nurses carry out roles that were traditionally those of doctors.
- *What other qualities, if any, might a nurse need in today's healthcare settings?* Although many of the qualities listed are probably still relevant to the twenty-first century, a nurse in today's NHS would need a much greater degree of skill and knowledge than in 1946, as treatments, decision making, technology and roles and responsibilities are all profoundly different. He or she would not be expected to work uncritically or with the degree of subservience required of the St George's Probationer.

1.5 Professional courtesy (page 13)

There are no fixed answers to these questions, but even as a student nurse you should expect to see basic standards of courtesy upheld by professionals; if not; you should talk to your university tutor about appropriate courses of action. The *NMC Code of Professional Conduct* (2008) gives definitive standards for professional courtesy and behaviour, to safeguard patients and the public. It is available at www.nmc-uk.org.

1.7 Service boundaries (pages 15–16)

- Acute emergency care following a heart attack would take place in an Emergency Department of a large acute sector NHS hospital.
- Long-term care of the elderly in nursing homes would normally take place in the private sector, in private residential and nursing homes. These may be paid for by the individual client and/or social services.
- Nursery provision for pre-school children with learning difficulties might take place in local authority settings or within other existing local nursery provision.
- Counselling and support of clients with alcohol and drug dependencies may take place within the NHS mental health system or might be undertaken by private and/or charity bodies.
- Hospice services for the terminally ill are normally provided by specific charities and are frequently linked to, but not part of, NHS hospitals.

Knowledge review

Having completed the chapter, how would you now rate your knowledge of the following topics?

	Good	Adequate	Poor
1. How was healthcare organised in Britain before the NHS?			
2. Why was the NHS born?			
3. How did the NHS develop?			
4. What are the benefits of the independent sector in healthcare?			
5. How developed is your appreciation of the relationship between management and clinicians in your current placement area?			

Further reading

Klein, R (2006) *The New Politics of the NHS,* 5th edition. London: Longman.
This is an essential text for those hoping to develop their knowledge of the recent history of the NHS.

Marsland, D (1996) *Welfare or Welfare State?* Basingstoke: Macmillan.
Examines issues of welfare state spending from a critical perspective.

Rivett, GC (1998) *From Cradle to Grave: Fifty years of the NHS,* online edition. London: King's Fund.
Available online at www.nhshistory.net/index.html (accessed 8 February 2007).

Useful websites

www.bbc.co.uk/history/british/modern/field_01.shtml BBC history site that looks briefly at the development of 'welfare' from early years to the present.
www.dh.gov.uk Department of Health website with comprehensive information about policy development, structures and organisational issues, including how policy developments differ in the UK countries. This should be consulted regularly when policies and legislation are announced.
www.nhs.uk/england/aboutTheNHS/history/default.cmsx NHS site that talks about the history of the NHS.
www.nhs.history.com The NHS history site, run by Geoffrey Rivett.

Chapter 2

Contemporary issues in healthcare policy

Chapter aims

After reading this chapter, you will able to outline:

- an overview of the development of the NHS since 1997;
- the influence and importance of the independent sector in contemporary healthcare;
- an awareness of how nurses' roles have developed in this period and of the different roles currently existing within nursing.

Introduction

Having examined in the previous chapter the establishment of the NHS, in this chapter we will examine key recent organisational and policy developments since 1997, current NHS structures and functions, the influence of the independent sector in healthcare, and the impact of contemporary policy on nurses.

Early policy promises

The Labour Party in opposition were highly critical of the politically motivated changes of successive Conservative governments and, when elected to power in 1997, initiated a series of changes designed to have considerable impact on patients, nurses and the organisation of the NHS. A theme of 'modernisation' was established and the initial rhetoric was to restore the NHS as a co-operative rather than the 'competitive' service they claimed it had become. The 1997 Labour Party Election Manifesto promised a new approach for the organisation of the NHS for nurses and patients – a critical opposition party outlining its vision for reform. The head-line statement was *We will save the NHS*. New Labour asserted that if the Conservatives were elected there would not be an NHS in five years' time, and that the 1990 NHS and Community Care Act had imposed a competitive internal market that strangled the NHS with costly and bureaucratic 'red tape'. Labour promised to increase spending on the NHS in real terms, with the money going towards patient care.

Hutton (1996) believed that Britain required a political route between an aggressive market-driven approach and a 'tax-and-spend' state-control approach. New Labour called this 'the third way', stating that for the NHS there was to be no return to the central control of the 1970s (Illiffe and Munro, 1997), but no abandoning of the central thrusts of Conservative policy such as quality improvement and consumerism. Policies for the NHS epitomised Labour's 'third way': the internal market and GP fund holding were ended, but the division between purchasers and providers of services was maintained, with health authorities paying for services and hospital and Primary Care Trusts (PCTs) providing them. In healthcare education, a similar system exists whereby higher education institutions tender for education contracts from health authorities, account for the services they provide in contract review meetings and involve service stakeholders in curriculum design.

The key concept in the NHS post-1997 was *modernization* (Klein, 2006), and a range of developments reflected this. For example, there was a new emphasis on using new technologies and the internet to improve access to healthcare for patients, and on using research findings and evidence-based practice so that professionals could be confident that what they do is informed by a current and appropriate knowledge base (McSherry and Haddock, 1999). 'Clinical governance' provides a forum for evaluation of these ideas, monitoring of standards and managing staff performance in clinical practice. Clinical governance was introduced as a means of ensuring accountability and quality in service provision (DH, 1998b), and is defined as a framework in which NHS organisations are accountable for continuously safeguarding and developing the quality of their services to ensure excellence (Scally and Donaldson, 1998). It covers a variety of activities (Clinical Governance Support Team, 2008), including:

- patient, public and carer involvement;
- risk management;
- staff management;
- education, training and continuous professional development;
- clinical effectiveness;
- information management;
- internal and external communication;
- leadership, including clinicians and management;
- team working.

Continuity *and* change were promised. Primary care was to continue its lead role, with GPs and nurses combining to plan more efficient local services. Higher-quality standards were promised for the acute sector hospital trusts, with more local accountability for trust management boards. However, despite the 1997 election rhetoric of change, Blakemore (1998, p189) described the health policies of Labour and Conservatives as *synchronised swimming* because of their similarity.

Elsewhere, the rhetoric concerned valuing and supporting staff. Recruitment, retention and fair pay were highlighted, and a new flexibility in working practices was hinted at, promising a 'new deal' (Boult and Allen, 1997), particularly for nurses.

The new NHS

A keystone of Labour health policy for England was the White Paper, *The New NHS – Modern, Dependable* (DH, 1997), with similar plans published for Scotland, Wales and Northern Ireland. This restated the founding principles of the NHS as a free service, based on need rather than the ability to pay. As of 1 April 1999, the internal market ended although the purchaser–provider split continued with a new emphasis on co-operation and 'integrated care', rather than on competition. GP fund holding was replaced by primary care groups. Here, large numbers of GPs combined to manage budgets for their patients' services, thus ending the Conservative internal market reforms, which had been criticised for being the first steps towards privatisation (Klein, 2006), ineffective at improving efficiency (Illiffe and Munro, 1997), and ineffectual in changing the culture of the NHS or convincing staff of their worth (Harrison et al., 1992).

Setting and monitoring standards was also to be a central theme for the NHS, and *The NHS Plan* (DH, 2000) introduced National Service Frameworks (NSFs) to set minimum standards and expectations for key service areas in health, in order to drive up standards for all. The key service areas are:

- coronary heart disease;
- cancer;

- paediatric intensive care;
- mental health;
- older people;
- diabetes;
- long-term conditions (LTCs);
- kidney disease;
- children;
- chronic obstructive pulmonary disease.

A further central element in the new NHS was the National Institute for Health and Clinical Excellence (NICE). This was originally established in 1999 as an independent organisation with responsibility for providing national guidance on the promotion of good health, and the prevention and treatment of ill health, to make sure that there is equal and consistent access to new treatments and procedures across the NHS. Its role was expanded to encompass guidance on public health, health technologies and clinical practice, including decisions concerning whether to allow controversial or expensive new drug treatments to be prescribed in the NHS and making sure that drug treatments are available to all rather than only to some in a 'postcode lottery' (NICE, 2005). The role of NICE and cost-effectiveness is discussed in more detail in Chapter 6.

A new system of performance assessment for the NHS was also developed. In 2001, the Healthcare Commission was established and took on functions previously exercised by the Commission for Health Improvement, the Audit Commission and other bodies. The Healthcare Commission describes itself as the *health watchdog* for England and is responsible for inspecting and monitoring standards in a range of areas, including safety, cleanliness and waiting times. The main aims of the Healthcare Commission are to: inspect NHS healthcare and public health provision for quality and value for money; keep the patients and the public informed with the best possible information about healthcare provision; and promote improvements where necessary (Healthcare Commission, 2008). It has a statutory duty to assess the performance of healthcare organisations, and awards annual performance ratings for the NHS in the form of a star rating system, known as the annual health checks (which can be accessed via their website at www.healthcarecommission.org.uk). For patients, a new Patient Advisory and Liaison service was established to provide help, advice and support for patients and their relatives, and a Patient Forum to allow a voice for patients in the way in which services were run. New national patient satisfaction surveys were also commissioned, to access patients' satisfaction with a variety of services (Klein, 2006).

Our healthier nation

In the light of the lack of success of the previous government's public health strategy, *The Health of the Nation*, the Labour government introduced *Saving Lives: Our healthier nation* (DH, 1999a) as an action plan to tackle poor health. The stated aims were to:

- improve the health of the general population;
- make significant improvements to the health of the poorest.

Like that of the Conservatives, Labour's new policy focused on the key illnesses of cancer, coronary heart disease and stroke, accidents and mental illness, but more specific targets were introduced, with progress towards meeting them monitored up until a completion date of 2010. Agencies including the NHS were thus charged with reducing:

- the cancer death rate in people under 75 by at least a fifth;
- the coronary heart disease and stroke death rate in people under 75 by at least two-fifths;
- the accident death rate by at least a fifth and serious injury by at least a tenth;
- the mental illness death rate from suicide and undetermined injury by at least a fifth.

In order to achieve this, the government pledged to alter the emphasis on service delivery towards tackling inequalities in health caused by poverty, low incomes and standards of living, so that individuals are empowered to make healthier choices about their own behaviour and lifestyles. Government promised to put in £21 billion for the NHS alone to help secure a healthier population, take action on smoking as the single biggest preventable cause of poor health, integrate central government and local government to work towards improving health, and emphasise health improvement and high standards for all citizens. The NHS was tasked with focusing on health improvement, and health authorities were to have a new role in improving the health of local people, with primary care groups and PCTs to have new responsibilities for public health. Local authorities were also asked to work in partnership with the NHS to plan for health improvement, by implementing health action zones and healthy living centres.

These targets were updated in an attempt to reduce the health gaps between rich and poor in the policy document *Tackling Health Inequalities: A programme for action* (DH, 2003b).

Activity 2.1

In order to begin to understand issues around smoking cessation, weight loss and their local provision, work through the exercises linked to the short scenario below.

Sally Smith is a friend of yours. She has two children at school and lives with her husband in a terraced house. With her last pregnancy she put on three stones in weight, and it is making her unhappy. She smokes 20 cigarettes a day and is desperate to stop because she realises the harm that she is doing to herself and to her children through passive smoking.

Activity 2.1 continued

- Sally knows that you are training to be a nurse and wants you to support her in her desire for change. How would you help Sally to change her lifestyle?
  - What practical advice could you offer her about losing weight and stopping smoking?
  - What health benefits would you tell her would accrue from stopping smoking? And from losing weight?
  - Search the internet for resources that might help you to support her, such as NHS smoking cessation information, and weight loss and diet advice.
- Investigate what services might be available to Sally in your local area.
  - Ask at your GP practice and the local leisure centre what facilities they might have to help people with smoking cessation and weight loss.
  - Ask at the local hospital if they have any facilities for outpatients.
  - Search the internet to see if there are any facilities provided locally by private companies. Compare their charges with those provided by the NHS and local authority leisure centres.

A brief outline of what you might discover is at the end of the chapter.

Widening access to healthcare

A new 24-hour helpline staffed by nurses called NHS Direct (www.nhsdirect.nhs.uk) was established in 1997. It proved popular in its initial pilots (DH, 1999c) and was extended to the whole country. It is a proactive service operating by referring callers to appropriate services out of hours; calling people who may need help; giving online health information on the internet and widening access; and publishing a reference guide to common illnesses for callers and for training. The intention was to give greater access to health information and support, and to make using services much easier (DH, 1999c).

In addition, a network of local health drop-in centres known as NHS Walk-in Centres has been established, intended to suit today's busy lifestyles. These cater for minor illnesses, freeing up GPs' time, and meaning that some patients can avoid long waits in accident and emergency (A & E) departments. These centres are staffed by doctors and nurses, working in tandem with traditional services. At the same time, GP out-of-hours services have been contracted to special companies, meaning that many GPs will no longer work substantial hours in their daily practice and then be required to cover emergencies at night.

Finances

When newly in power, the Labour government initially maintained health spending within the limits set by their Conservative predecessors, but *Working Together* (NHS Executive, 1998c) committed an extra £21 billion in spending over three years. This spending was conditional on achieving targets in key areas such as modernisation. Sir Derek Wanless, a former Chief Executive of the National Westminster Bank, produced a report (Wanless, 2002) indicating that, throughout the 1980s and 1990s, the NHS had been underfunded, falling short of the European average figures. As a result there was an unprecedented growth in spending on the NHS from 1997 to 2005, with the budget promised to rise to £92 billion by 2008 (Klein, 2006), as the government sought to increase health spending to about 9–10 per cent of gross domestic product (GDP – a measure of the size of a country's economy, being the total value of all the goods and services produced in a year), to match European averages (Wanless et al., 2007).

In order to increase the amount of funding available for building projects and facilities, a scheme was introduced to the health sector called the private finance initiative (PFI). This allowed private companies to invest money in building NHS sites (as they did in other areas such as schools). When completed, the new hospitals would be owned and run by the private contractor, with the NHS paying to lease the facilities and services from the company on 30-year contracts, after which the company would own the site. The government saw these arrangements as a means of renewing the antiquated NHS estate without spending tax revenues, and of delivering a high-quality service on time to specified standards (HM Treasury, 2007). From 1997 to 2007, 80 sites had major PFI work planned, in progress or completed at a cost of over £16 billion pounds, compared to six sites having major publicly funded work, at a cost of £500 million (DH, 2007c, d). However, despite the huge sums of money made available for NHS building projects under PFI, critics of the scheme argue that it does not work in the best interests of NHS patients and staff, that it has not always resulted in value for money, and that there has been little or no protection for the NHS if things go wrong (McGauran, 2002).

Nursing received special financial attention, with a £5 million recruitment advertising campaign to attract qualified nurses back into the profession. An extra £23 million was allocated to ensure *a new, enhanced role for nurses in the 21st century* (DH, 1998a), particularly in areas such as extending nurse prescribing. There was a £5 million increase on the non-means tested bursary for students, and £4 million extra for 'return to practice' courses (which facilitate nurses who have been out of the workplace for years to acquire the necessary skills to function in today's NHS).

NHS Foundation Trusts, Primary Care Trusts and Strategic Health Authorities

The Health and Social Care Community Health and Standards Act (2003) established NHS Foundation Trusts as 'public benefit' corporations, a new type of non-profit making organisation with more independence than had been the case in the NHS, where previously there was a high degree of central control from the DH. With NHS Foundation Trusts the Secretary of State has no such power of direction, the intention being to allow them to relate more directly to their local stakeholders in service provision, particularly patients and the local community. NHS Foundation Trusts must have membership of their Management Boards elected from among their local populations (DH, 2000). While there has been criticism that establishing Foundation Trusts might create a two-tier NHS as other non-Foundation Trusts were left behind, the DH maintains that they continue to operate within NHS principles such as free care based on need, not ability to pay (DH, 2007a). It is intended that all Trusts will gain Foundation status if they are able to do so.

NHS Foundation Trusts enjoy greater licence than other NHS Trusts, such as:

- freedom from central control and performance management by Strategic Health Authorities;
- freedom to access capital (money) at Trust level rather than the current system of central allocation;
- freedom to invest surpluses in developing new local services;
- local flexibility to tailor new governance arrangements to their communities.

The Healthcare Commission inspects NHS Foundation Trusts, just like other Trusts, but they are also overseen by an independent regulator called Monitor, which has considerable powers to intervene if there are major management or financial problems. The first NHS Foundation Trusts were authorised in 2004, and by 2007 there were 54 in operation (DH, 2007a).

Health Reform in England: Update and next steps (DH, 2006a) outlined a framework for taking forward the reform of the NHS, with:

- more choice and a much stronger voice for patients;
- money following patients, rewarding the best and most efficient providers, thus giving others the incentive to improve;
- more diverse providers, with more freedom to innovate and improve services;
- a framework of system management, regulation and decision making that guarantees safety and quality, fairness, equity and value for money (Carruthers, 2006).

These ideas informed the reorganisation of Primary Care Trusts (PCTs) and Strategic Health Authorities (SHAs) in 2007. The functions of these bodies are as follows.

A PCT exists to (DH, 2006b):

- engage with its local population to improve health and well-being;
- commission a comprehensive and equitable range of high-quality, responsive and efficient services, within allocated resources, and contract for services with other NHS Trusts and private providers;
- provide high-quality, responsive and efficient services where this gives best value for money. Primary care providers are GPs, dentists, opticians, pharmacists, NHS walk-in centres, NHS Direct and care trusts;

- be directly accountable to their local population and to SHAs. PCTs operate within the framework of DH policy; they are held to account for this by SHAs, not directly by the Department (DH, 2007b).

A Strategic Health Authority exists to (DH, 2006b):

- give strategic leadership in healthcare;
- provide organisational and workforce development;
- ensure local systems operate effectively and deliver improved performance; their relationships and accountability should encompass (DH, 2006b):
- partnership working with their PCTs and regional organisations, particularly Government Offices for the Regions;
- holding PCTs to account for their performance;
- being held to account by the DH for ensuring their local health systems operate effectively and in line with government policy.

Numbers of SHAs were reduced from 28 to 10 in a major reconfiguration of roles in July 2006 in England, in an attempt to improve service quality and generate financial savings.

Patient power and patient choice are central to the new NHS, with patients to be given greater opportunity to choose where they are treated, and by which hospitals, by 2008 (Klein, 2006). There is also to be a new emphasis on partnership working between the NHS and independent and voluntary sectors, with the NHS funding activity and treatment for its patients in these sectors. In addition to hospital and primary care provision within the NHS, a new *policy revolution* (Klein, 2006) initiated the establishment of 'stand-alone' diagnostic and surgical treatment centres (called independent treatment centres), where patients could be referred for many kinds of surgery. These are run largely by private companies in the independent sector, but with operations paid for from NHS funds. By 2005 there were 32 of these, doing about 10 per cent of elective NHS operations (Klein, 2006).

An Act of Parliament, called the Health Act 2006 (DH, 2006c), made a variety of changes to the law to support the issues discussed above, simplifying some aspects and restating others. A smoking ban in most public places was also introduced in July 2007. A code of practice was issued for controlling healthcare-associated infection.

The impact on nurses

Nurses were promised new areas of contribution to patient care, outlined in a key policy document called *Making a Difference: Strengthening the nursing, midwifery and health visiting contribution to health and health care* (DH, 1999b). Its theme was 'more', and it included promises to improve education, training and working conditions, leading to more satisfying careers.

Throughout, it was argued that nurses faced new challenges in the future and that structures existing at the time often constrained nurses' ability to innovate: if these structures were loosened, nurses could begin to work in new, more innovative ways. They were asked to raise their expectations and, supported by new technology, to contribute in a variety of new roles (*The NHS Plan*, DH, 2000). A range of ideas was developed to allow nurses to contribute to patient care in innovative ways. There would be:

- more qualified nurses and 'return to nursing' opportunities;
- more flexible opportunities for education and training, with a restructuring of pre-registration training (UKCC, 1999) and an emphasis on practice skills and practice support;
- new career structures with progression linked to responsibilities and competencies and the end of clinical grading;
- an improvement in working lives (NHS Executive, 1998c) with a greater emphasis on equality, staff involvement and healthy workplaces;
- strengthening leadership, with a new emphasis on ward management leadership development, underpinned by the return of the title Matron to denote a new senior nurse role, and Nurse Consultants;
- modernisation of professional self-regulation: the United Kingdom Central Council for Nursing and Midwifery (UKCC) was replaced by the Nursing and Midwifery Council (NMC), which continues to be the statutory body charged with holding registration of nurses, midwives and health visitors, and maintaining and ensuring practitioner standards;
- working in new ways: roles for nurses were to be extended to make better use of skills (such as prescribing medications); nurse-led primary care services were to improve access and responsiveness; there was to be careful monitoring of innovative roles; and the quality of care was to be enhanced (DH, 1998b).

In addition, a major review of pay and conditions in the NHS was undertaken. This was known as *Agenda for Change* (DH, 2007e), and these recommendations were implemented on 1 December 2004. All jobs, including those of nurses, were profiled in a process known as 'job evaluation', and staff were then 'slotted into' a new banding structure, based on the *NHS Knowledge and Skills Framework* (KSF). The KSF was developed as part of the Agenda for Change process to update the definition of NHS posts and to allow for progression and development within the service based on demonstrating achievement of particular competencies (or 'dimensions'). The KSF lays out clearly the knowledge and skills that NHS staff need in order to deliver quality services (RCN, 2005a).

The six core dimensions for every NHS job are:

- communication;
- personal and people development;
- health, safety and security;
- service development;
- quality;
- equality, diversity and rights.

There are a further 24 specific dimensions in four categories that can be applied to define parts of different posts (these are health and well-being, information and knowledge, general, and estates and facilities). Each dimension has four levels, called 'indicators'. The higher the level (4 is highest), the greater the expectation of the level of knowledge and skills necessary for a post (RCN, 2005a).

Many nurses welcomed Agenda for Change and the KSF. The proposals were discussed and negotiated in agreement with professional bodies, including the Royal

College of Nursing (RCN). However, on implementation they were not universally popular. In many areas staff were required to reapply for jobs that they had been doing for years, and in many cases nurses were made redundant or did not go into the band that they might have expected (for more information on this and the NHS KSF, see the RCN website at www.rcn.org.uk/agendaforchange). Qualified nurses' bands begin at Band 5 (replacing the previous clinical D grade). A Band 6 would be a more senior nurse such as a 'junior sister'; Band 7 would be a specialist nurse or a Matron; and Band 8 a Senior Matron or Nurse Consultant (although these job titles are not universal and some Trusts and PCTs use other titles).

At the same time as Agenda for Change, there is a new drive to reduce the numbers of Band 5 nurses and establish a new skill mix with the introduction of 'assistant practitioner' roles at Band 4. These nurses are trained in more vocational two-year foundation degrees rather than the traditional three-year diploma and degree programmes. They are not 'registered nurses' with the NMC as Band 5 staff nurses would be, but provide a level of proficient hands-on care in support of Band 5 nurses. There will be fewer registered practitioners of Band 5 and above in healthcare, but they will be expected to undertake more specialist and technical activities, with increased leadership aspects to their roles. This means that qualified nurses of Band 5 and above can expect to carry greater responsibilities than previously with appropriate post-registration training; for example, being responsible for admitting and discharging patients independently, diagnosing and initiating treatments, and prescribing medications. Roles previously undertaken by doctors alone are increasingly likely to be carried out by nurses; evidence suggests that patients generally approve of this and receive a good quality of service as a result (see, for example, Moore, 1998; Williamson et al., 2007).

Thus, New Labour's changes generally offer greater scope and opportunity for nurses, as they are now able to move into new areas of responsibility for patient care. While not new, roles such as Advanced Practitioner and Clinical Specialist have increased in number; for example, a survey for the RCN found that three-quarters of Nurse Practitioners had been responsible in setting up their own posts (Ball, 2006).

CASE STUDY

Jane is a Nurse Practitioner in the Emergency Department of the local NHS Foundation Trust. She qualified initially as a staff nurse with a Bachelor of Science (BSc Honours) in Adult Nursing with NMC registration from a large cohort of students at the university. Her first job was as a Band 5 staff nurse on a surgical ward, where she stayed for two years, completing her preceptorship, consolidating her skills and confidence, and becoming familiar with the role of a qualified nurse. After two years, she moved to a job on the coronary care unit because she wanted to gain some 'medical' experience as well as gain knowledge and skills in more acute care settings. After one year, the opportunity came for her to move again, this time to the Emergency Department. She really enjoyed the pace and variety of emergency nursing, and decided that this was where she wanted to specialise and carry on her career.

CASE STUDY CONTINUED

After three years working in the department, where she gained a wide variety of clinical and managerial skills, Jane secured promotion to Band 6 as a Sister, with responsibility for the minor injuries area of the department. After a further year, the senior clinical staff in the department were tasked with reviewing the services provided, with a specific remit to investigate how the contribution of senior nursing staff such as Jane could better be utilised. It was decided to create a number of Nurse Practitioner roles within the department. These posts were intended to improve patient care and service delivery by giving these nurses greater autonomy in decision making so that they could see patients independently, make diagnoses, initiate clinical investigations and treatments, and take responsibility for admissions and discharges. Jane was offered the opportunity to undertake further study in order to equip her for her new role and she was supported by her Trust to enrol on a Master's degree (MSc) in Advanced Nursing Practice at the university, which was accredited by the RCN (2005b). This programme included modules on leadership and management skills, patient assessment and diagnostic clinical skills, consultation skills, nurse prescribing and research methods. She was fortunate in that she received good support from medical staff in the department, and was able to increase her knowledge, skills and confidence.

Jane was pleased with her new role. She could see that she was making a difference to patient care and service delivery. She had felt frustrated in her Sister's role before she became a Nurse Practitioner, because, although she had an excellent knowledge base and clinical skills in emergency care and could do her job well, she was still required to gain approval and consent from junior doctors in the department, some of whom had very limited experience of emergency care and were still in training themselves.

While she made an effort to get on with everybody that she worked with and usually did so, there were times when she knew what to do for patients, but the constant need, for example, to gain junior doctors' signatures on prescriptions for analgesics or on X-ray request forms, in her opinion hindered diagnosis and treatment, left patients in unnecessary pain and suffering, and slowed down patient throughput in the department because patients waited longer to see a doctor after already seeing a nurse.

Jane always had the support of medical staff and was able to refer to them when she was unable to help patients herself, if they were too sick or if she was unsure about diagnoses or treatments. In her new role as Nurse Practitioner, and equipped with the appropriate advanced clinical and prescribing skills, she was able to act with greater autonomy as a key clinical decision maker in the department. When the department audited its waiting times and patient satisfaction rates, it was shown that the new Nurse Practitioner roles speeded up diagnosis, treatment and discharge, and that patients were very satisfied with the new service. On completion of the MSc, Jane was able to gain a Band 7 post as an emergency department Nurse Practitioner.

In order to begin to appreciate how a career in nursing might develop, and the additional roles and responsibilities that a specialist nurse might undertake, read the case study above and work through the following.

- Use the internet to search for information on these new roles within nursing:
  - Modern Matrons;
  - Ward Managers;
  - Clinical Specialists;
  - Nurse Consultants;
  - Nurse Practitioners.

A brief outline of what you might find is at the end of the chapter.

- Write a brief job description of each role based on DH websites and information you might find from relevant organisations such as the RCN.

- Identify and approach members of staff in these roles in your own organisations; politely ask them about their roles and their daily responsibilities. Compare these conversations with the information you collected in the first two questions above.

New Labour's NHS legacy

In May 2007 Tony Blair stepped aside as Prime Minister after ten years. Bearing in mind that in 1997 New Labour promised to *save the NHS*, what was his legacy? Writing in the *British Medical Journal* (*BMJ*), Polly Toynbee (2007, p1031) put it thus:

> *This has been a decade of turmoil, with zigzag reforms dictated from the top, only to be countermanded again from the top. The history of his 'reforms' hardly bears repeating. First he dismantled general practice fundholding and some aspects of the Tory internal market. He set up primary care groups, remade them into primary care trusts, and then merged them again into half the number. Demolished regional health authorities were resurrected as 28 strategic health authorities and then merged again back into the original 10 regions . . . However often Tony Blair and his health ministers recite their litany of successes and improvements, public opinion heads downwards. Voters asked about the NHS said it was a disaster.*

Despite the impressive rhetoric of modernisation, patient choice, opportunities for staff and funding expansions, by 2007 NHS finances were in crisis and in many areas nurses were unable to secure jobs on qualification or were subject to redundancies, and training places were cut. This was blamed in part on a greatly increased wages bill, particularly for senior doctors (Klein, 2006), and partly on a new system of 'fixed pricing', meaning that Trusts received a fixed price for the services they provided, which were often not enough to cover the actual costs of service delivery (Lambert, 2007).

Others have criticised the New Labour government's reforms as being wasteful, costing approximately £3 billion to implement with only minimal impact, creating structures very similar to those set up by the previous Conservative government. There is evidence that many hospitals now delay operations in order to save money (Halligan, 2007a, b). Further questions hang over a new computer system managed by Connecting for Health, which is likely to cost billions of pounds more than expected and has so far failed to deliver the proposed outcomes; the NHS has also simply failed to deal with the issues of hospital-acquired infections or dangerous multi-resistant bacteria (Toynbee, 2007).

Sir Derek Wanless (Wanless et al., 2007) reviewed NHS spending and achievements in 2007. His report concluded that total UK spending on NHS care had increased to £113 billion for 2007/08, coming close to the European average, but, as this extra spending will tail off after 2008 to about 3 per cent per annum until 2010/11, the UK would once again be near the bottom of the European health-spending league. Doctors' and nurses' pay increases were blamed for increasing costs (the Agenda for Change reforms cost £1.8 billion), and Wanless (Wanless et al., 2007) concludes that there is no evidence to suggest that significant benefits have resulted from this extra spending. Even so, as old buildings are replaced, new NHS facilities are opened and demand levels increase, there are unlikely to be enough staff and more will be required to cope with the increased activity levels; indeed, Wanless outlines how the NHS has had to do more in all areas as a result of its expansion. The founders of the NHS might recognise this paradox: with more capacity comes more demand, which in turn requires a greater investment of resources to cope. On policy, Wanless et al. (2007) give cautious approval to the direction in which government policy has moved, particularly the emphasis on organisational change and service redesign, but find that there is insufficient evidence to indicate whether these changes have been successful at this point. They conclude that costs will continue to rise: without significant increases in productivity in the whole NHS, and without major public health successes such as 'winning the battle against obesity', it is likely the NHS will become expensive – so costly, in fact, that taxes would have to rise to such a high level as to undermine its current popularity.

Information point

This chapter and the preceding one have only dealt with key legislation and policies on the NHS and health. So much has been done by every post-war government that it is not possible, nor even desirable that, at this stage, a student nurse should understand it all in detail. While governments continue to decide health policy and take such direct control of the service through the DH, the NHS will remain a 'political football' and a large part of the battleground at election times. For staff working in the NHS, change is a

Information point continued

constant factor, which at times leaves them feeling like part of a *permanent revolution*, according to the Secretary of State for Health, Alan Johnson (2007).

In all the above discussion of key legislation and policy changes it is worth knowing that the policies discussed in this and the preceding chapter are primarily about England. Specific details of arrangements for England, Scotland, Wales and Northern Ireland in all the policy developments discussed above can be found at www.dh.gov.uk/, and for the full text of Acts of Parliament, see www.opsi.gov.uk/. Although overarching principles were similar for Scotland, Northern Ireland, England and Wales, details and structures created were slightly different throughout the UK. This has been the case throughout the history of the NHS, and this tendency for separate implementation of policy has accelerated as Scotland, Wales and Northern Ireland have gained their own elected governments.

Scotland has had some devolved government powers, including making its own laws on health since the Scotland Act 1998 (for further information, visit the Scottish Parliament website at www.scottish.parliament.uk/home.htm).

The Welsh assembly was established following the Government of Wales Act 1998. It has had the power to make its own laws for health since the Government of Wales Act 2006 (see the Welsh Assembly website at www.wales.gov.uk/).

The picture is more complex in Northern Ireland because, although re-established after the Northern Ireland (Elections) Act in 1998, the Northern Ireland Assembly was suspended several times until 2007, when devolved powers were restored. During periods of suspension, power reverted to the UK Parliament's Northern Ireland Office. Northern Ireland now has a Department of Social Security and Public Safety, and the assembly has legislative powers for health and health services (for more information, see www.niassembly.gov.uk/).

CHAPTER SUMMARY

- Despite criticising the outgoing Conservative government's policies, following their election in 1979 the incoming Labour government continued much of the direction, with an emphasis on reform and modernisation.
- New Labour policy still looks like an 'internal market', as GPs commission services, with a high degree of choice for patients and money following patients to successful Trusts; and there are more service providers than simply the state's NHS.
- Key organisational developments were the introduction of NHS Foundation Trusts, a continuation of the emphasis on community health and lifestyle provision, a pay and conditions review for all staff, and the reconfiguration of health authorities and PCTs.

- The basic structure of the NHS remains, with primary and secondary care, but with a much greater emphasis on service provision in primary care, and a reduction in numbers of SHAs from 28 to 10 in England.
- New facilities such as walk-in centres and NHS Direct have widened access to services; the independent sector now makes a contribution for NHS patients by providing some surgical care in treatment centres.
- For nurses there have been opportunities to develop their skills and roles, and a new career structure has been established.
- Although activity levels have increased, these reforms have been costly and, some argue, financially wasteful, with little evidence of success in many areas, or of long-term sustainability.
- These are important ideas for nurses to understand as they are the context in which contemporary NHS provision operates.

Activities: brief outline answers

2.1 Sally Smith (pages 24–5)

How would you help Sally to change her lifestyle?
- *What practical advice could you offer her about losing weight and stopping smoking?* You should tell her to get help, as smoking cessation groups and weight loss groups have been shown to be beneficial compared to will-power alone.
- *What health benefits would you tell her would accrue from stopping smoking? And from losing weight?* You could inform her of the health benefits that she would find if she stopped smoking (reduction in risk of cancer, heart disease and chronic lung problems) and lost weight (reduction in risk of diabetes and heart disease). You might add that there are risks to her children from passive smoking, and calculate the money she would save from not buying cigarettes every day. At about £5 per packet per day she could save £1,825 in a year!
- *Search the internet for resources that might help you to support her, such as NHS smoking cessation information, and weight loss and diet advice.* These should be accessible in your local area.

Investigate what services might be available to Sally in your local area.
- *Ask at your GP practice and the local leisure centre what facilities they might have to help people with smoking cessation and weight loss.* GP practices should have information about local smoking cessation sessions, and GPs can refer people for exercise classes at the leisure centre, which are on prescription and free. GPs may prescribe nicotine replacement products. The leisure centre may run its own smoking cessation groups, and will have exercise facilities offering training on equipment, structure and support.
- *Ask at the local hospital if they have any facilities for outpatients.* The local hospital may offer smoking cessation.
- *Search the internet to see if there are any facilities provided locally by private companies. Compare their charges with those provided by the NHS and local*

authority leisure centres. The answers you find to this will depend on what is available locally. Boots the Chemist offer a free smoking cessation service, and hypnotherapists will treat smokers for a charge. Some nicotine replacement products are available over the counter. Pharmacists will provide advice about suitable products.

2.2 New roles (page 32)

- *Modern Matrons.* This term was introduced to give patients a clear authority figure. Although initially a senior nurse with wide responsibility for a directorate or service, now Ward Managers are Matrons, and Modern Matrons are Senior Matrons in many Trusts.
- *Ward Managers.* Once known as Sister, a Ward Manager (often now called a Matron) has day-to-day, 24-hour responsibility for care standards and a team of nurses in a ward or department.
- *Clinical Specialists.* This is a specialist nurse with clinical responsibility for a group of patients, such as cystic fibrosis patients, or procedures such as endoscopy.
- *Nurse Consultants.* These are new, very senior nurses, with wide-ranging responsibilities for clinical care, service management and delivery, teaching and research. They will have a very high degree of autonomy and work in partnership with doctors.
- *Nurse Practitioners.* These nurses have clinical responsibilities for groups of patients, and will have additional clinical skills that other nurses do not have, for example diagnostic and prescribing skills, gained through experience and additional qualifications. They will have a high degree of autonomy in defined areas, such as Emergency Department nursing.

Knowledge review

Having completed the chapter, how would you now rate your knowledge of the following topics?

	Good	Adequate	Poor
1. How has the NHS developed since 1997?			
2. What is the influence and importance of the independent sector in contemporary healthcare?			
3. What new roles have been established for nurses in recent times?			
4. What provision is there in your locality for facilitating smoking cessation and weight loss?			

Further reading

Hart, C (2004) *Nurses and Politics: The impact of power and practice.* Basingstoke: Palgrave Macmillan.
This is a useful text that outlines some of the impact of NHS change on nurses and nursing.

Klein, R (2006) *The New Politics of the NHS,* 5th edition. London: Longman.
This is an essential text for those hoping to develop their knowledge of the recent history of the NHS.

Dodds, S, Chamberlain, C and Williamson, GR (2006) Modernizing chronic obstructive pulmonary disease admissions to improve patient care: local outcomes from implementing the Ideal Design of Emergency Access project. *Accident and Emergency Nursing* 14: 141–7.
An example of a successful modernisation project.

Dodds, S and Williamson, GR (2007) Nurse-led arterial blood gas sampling for patients requiring long term oxygen therapy. *Nursing Times Respiratory Supplement* 103(44).
An example of the roles nurses are now able to undertake that had previously been undertaken only by doctors. Available online at www.nursingtimes.net/nursingtimes/pages/DevelopmentNurseLedarterialbloodgassamplingforpatients.

Toynbee, P (2007) NHS: the Blair years. *British Medical Journal* 334: 1030–1.
Available online at http://bmj.com/cgi/content/full/334/7602/1030.

Williamson, GR, Collinson, S and Withers, N (2007) Patient satisfaction audit of a nurse-led lung cancer follow-up clinic. *Cancer Nursing Practice*, 6(8): 31–5.
An example of the establishment of a nurse-led service in lung cancer.

Useful websites

www.dh.gov.uk Department of Health website with comprehensive information about policy development, structures and organisational issues. Search here also for NSF information.

www.gosmokefree.co.uk NHS website with information and resources to help someone stop smoking.

www.healthcarecommission.org.uk Healthcare Commission site for more information on performance indicators and rating scales.

www.nhsdirect.nhs.uk NHS direct website with many relevant resources, including weight loss advice.

www.nhshistory.com The NHS history site, run by Geoffrey Rivett.

www.nhsu.nhs.uk/ksf/index.html NHS KSF Advisory Service, which has been established to provide support to individuals and managers using the *NHS Knowledge and Skills Framework* (KSF).

www.nice.org.uk National Institute for Health and Clinical Excellence website.

www.opsi.gov.uk Office of Public Sector Information. This site can be searched for full details of Acts of Parliament.

www.rcn.org.uk Royal College of Nursing (RCN): the professional association for nurses. Similar in some respects to a trade union.

www.rcn.org.uk/agendaforchange For information on *Agenda for Change* and the NHS KSF.

www.rdehospital.nhs.uk/rde/rde.htm Royal Devon and Exeter NHS Foundation Trust. Navigate around the site for examples of the variety of activities undertaken by an NHS Foundation Trust.

www.skills forhealth.org.uk/ksfcomps.php Skills for Health site for mapping NHS KSF competencies to current roles.

Chapter 3

Nursing, policy making and politics

NMC Standards of Proficiency

This chapter will address the following NMC *Standards of Proficiency* and *Outcomes to be achieved for entry to the branch programme.*

Provide a rationale for the nursing care delivered which takes account of social, cultural, spiritual, legal, political and economic influences.

Demonstrate a commitment to the need for continuing professional development and personal supervision activities in order to enhance knowledge, skills, values and attitudes needed for safe and effective nursing practice.

Outcomes to be achieved for entry to the branch programme:
Demonstrate responsibility for one's own learning through the development of a portfolio of practice and recognise when further learning is required:

- identify specific learning needs and objectives;
- begin to engage with, and interpret, the evidence base which underpins nursing practice.

Acknowledge the importance of seeking supervision to develop safe and effective nursing practice.

Chapter aims

After reading this chapter you will be able to outline:

- how the registration of nursing evolved and how nurse education has developed recently;
- the roles of political parties, government and Parliament in shaping health policies;
- the role of the Chief Nursing Officer;
- how the press and television present health policy topics and influence the policy agenda;
- the roles of trade unions, the Royal College of Nursing (RCN) and the International Council of Nurses (ICN).

Introduction

In this chapter we will be looking at a variety of areas where politics, policy making and nursing practice intersect. We will begin by looking at how the law relating to nursing has changed over time. In the past, anyone could nurse but now nurses require registration, with strict control of entry standards to the nursing profession for qualified nurses through programmes of education, and clear standards of conduct and behaviour for practitioners who want to continue on the register and therefore practice as nurses. Next, we will look at some influences on political parties' health policies and their impact on government and Parliament. Then we will examine the media's influence on the health policy agenda, in the form of the press and of television reporting, using the specific examples of the NICE (2007) ruling on the treatment of Alzheimer's disease, and the Bristol Royal Infirmary Inquiry into their paediatric heart surgery services. Finally, we will look at the roles of trade unions and the RCN and their influence on health policy, and the role of the RCN as the nurses' professional body.

The evolution of registration for nurses

These days, nurses and nursing have a status in society and within healthcare organisations. This status, although not equal to that of doctors and medicine, is an indication of how nursing is viewed in society. However, nursing has not always had such a status. It has been a hard-fought battle to gain recognition for nursing and for it to be seen as a profession in the eyes of the public. Nowadays, UK nurses must complete recognised programmes of study, including theoretical components as well as practice placements, in order to gain degree and diploma qualifications leading to registration with the Nursing and Midwifery Council (NMC) as Band 5 registered practitioners. This registration is a legal requirement in order to practise as a nurse, in any branch and including midwifery and health visiting, and its roots go back into the nineteenth century.

Developing registration

The Victorians were concerned that nurses were not always morally virtuous. Their attempts to train nurses were bound in with the desire to improve the moral standing of nurses themselves. In the late nineteenth century and early twentieth century, this 'character building' strategy or 'domestic academy' model, beloved of Florence Nightingale (of whom we talk more in Chapter 4), was slowly overtaken by the idea that nursing should aim more for a professional status and a scientific approach borrowed from medicine. This new strategy and associated training was introduced by the nursing reformer Ethel Bedford Fenwick, Matron of St Bartholomew's Hospital, London (Rafferty, 1996). In 1887, Henry Burdett established the National Pension Fund for Nurses (NPFN), and had the idea of noting all trained nurses' names and experience in a public register, showing who qualified for Fund benefits. However, Burdett and Fenwick disagreed, Nightingale was set against registration in general, and the NPFN scheme failed to develop into a meaningful method of regulating nursing, partly because each hospital regarded its nurses as *its* nurses and believed that a central or state system would undermine this relationship.

Mrs Bedford Fenwick and her supporters formed the British Nurses' Association (BNA, which became the Royal British Nurses' Association (RBNA) in 1891), in an attempt to establish registration dependent on scientific training including medical and surgical knowledge, to bring about self-governance for nurses, and to guarantee the public's safety from incompetent or immoral nurses. This move was supported by the British Medical Association (BMA), which passed a resolution in 1895 calling for the registration of appropriately skilled and qualified nurses (White, 1976). When the RBNA applied to become the body responsible for registration, they were turned down, but in 1899 the International Council of Nurses (ICN) was established, partly to campaign for registration, and in 1902 the Society for State Registration of Nurses (SSRN) was set up to do the same (Rafferty, 1996). A Bill to establish registration for nurses came before Parliament each year from 1904 to 1914, but bringing it into legislation was evaded by government (Abel-Smith, 1960).

In the aftermath of World War I (WWI, which lasted from 1914 to 1918), the calls for registration were heeded. Trained nurses sought to distance themselves from the large numbers of untrained nurses who had become involved in caring for the war casualties, public sympathies for nurses ran high, and women finally gained the vote after serious campaigning by the Suffragettes. This combination of political pressures brought about change (Chapman, 1998). Consideration also began to be given to the future training and supply of nurses, as during WWI there were 220,000 military beds staffed by 12,000 trained nurses, but only about 6,000 nurses trained to look after the non-military sick (Abel-Smith, 1960).

In 1916, Arthur Stanley, Chairman of the British Red Cross Society, proposed a College of Nursing, similar to the Royal Colleges of Physicians and Surgeons. The College began in 1916 (later becoming the Royal College of Nursing, RCN), to promote better education and training for nurses, recognise approved training schools, maintain a register of appropriately qualified nurses, and to lobby Parliament in the interests of the nursing profession. Male and mental health nurses were excluded from membership. Agreement could not be found between the RBNA and the new College, and in 1919 an Act of Parliament (the Nurses Registration Act 1919) was passed, establishing a General Nursing Council (GNC) to register nurses, in four parts:

- a general part for all, and a supplementary part for male nurses;
- a part for mental health nurses;
- a part for sick children's nurses;
- and a last part for others.

Nurses without formal training could register if they could satisfy the Council that they were of good character and had three years' experience, but unqualified volunteer nurses (Voluntary Aid Detachments or VADs) were expressly not to gain registration in order to protect the jobs of 'properly qualified' nurses. The fee was one guinea. The Council would also approve training schools, and produced an advisory code for the syllabus to be followed in such establishments (Abel-Smith, 1960).

This development was hailed as the moment when nursing 'came of age' as a profession, emulating medicine (for which registration came in the 1858 Medical Act) and overtaking the law and the clergy in its ability to set standards, regulate entry and protect the public (Abel-Smith, 1960). In addition, nursing now began to take control of its education (Chapman, 1998), and, while the first Council was appointed (in 1920), thereafter it would be elected by those on the register. Although practising nurses could apply for admission to the new register until 1923, in 1925 the first nurses were admitted on the sole basis of new examinations, as the GNC established a 'single portal of entry' to the register based on three years' training in approved training schools. Attempts at introducing a second-level qualification were, at that time, firmly resisted.

A second-level qualification

However, by 1925 there were severe shortages of nurses, a situation that continued until the outbreak of WWII in 1938; in 1937 it was estimated that the entire output of girls from state secondary schools would be needed to meet the demand for nurses. Hospitals began to employ more 'orderlies' or assistant nurses – positions for those with a practical bent. They could be entered on a GNC 'roll' after 1939 following two years' training. This was a second level of qualification (Abel-Smith, 1960) and, in 1943, a Nurses Act was passed to legitimise the status of these assistant nurses (Rafferty, 1996).

Although bitterly opposed by some in the profession such as Mrs Bedford Fenwick, this move was portrayed as a cornerstone in the further professionalisation of nursing. If registered nurses were to be the leaders, then assistant nurses would help and support them in some of the less intellectually demanding ward tasks, leaving Probationers with more time for training under the direct supervision of registered nurses instead of carrying out those more basic duties (Abel-Smith, 1960).

Recent developments

Several Nurses Acts were passed between 1943 and 1979, and there were many reports and reorganisations during this period, but they focused on manpower issues rather than education, and their impacts were mostly relatively minor compared to the establishment of registration after 1919 (Chapman, 1989).

The Nurses, Midwives and Health Visitors Act (1979) provided a major reorganisation for training and registration, and influences contemporary nursing to this day. The 1979 Act followed the recommendations of the Briggs Committee (1972), providing a powerful national body in the United Kingdom Central Council for Nursing, Midwifery and Health Visiting (UKCC). This began in 1983, and oversaw the work of the National Boards for England, Scotland, Northern Ireland and Wales. The independent bodies that had previously controlled educational matters in those countries (Leathard, 2000) were replaced by the new UKCC so that post-1979 registration, education and standard setting were unified in a stronger national entity. The 1979 Act was amended by a 1992 Act, so that the principal functions of the UKCC were to:

- approve training institutions and ensure their content met the required standards;
- improve standards of training for nurses, midwives and health visitors, and make sure these met the requirements of the European Community;
- lay down the necessary conditions for entry to the register and for post-registration training;
- provide advice as to the required standards of conduct.

One major change that occurred with the 1992 Act was that the Boards of each country lost the ability to investigate professional misconduct, which became the responsibility of the UKCC. The Council continued as an elected body, with 40 members elected from practising nurses, and 20 appointed by government (Pyne, 1998).

Nurse education, higher education and purchasing consortia

Nurse education was relocated gradually throughout the 1990s from its previous base in NHS training hospitals into the higher education (HE) sector, mostly in the universities that were created post-1992 from what had previously been poly-technics, although some older universities do offer pre-registration programmes. This movement into HE was problematic for some teaching staff as the two sectors (HE and the NHS) were quite distinct in their organisation and ethos, and many nurse teachers with good records in clinical practice and clinical teaching found themselves in new institutions that often valued teaching and research skills above clinical practice. The move meant further changes as universities required academic validation of nurses' programmes of study, and often meant that lecturers had to teach larger groups than previously (Carlisle et al., 1996). For others, moving into the university sector offered great opportunities for professional advancement, as well as access to a range of facilities that the NHS could not have provided.

In the 1990s, government introduced a radical restructuring of the NHS (see Chapter 1). At the same time nurse education underwent a similar radical restructuring because of *Working for Patients* (DH, 1989), which contained *Working Paper 10: Education and training*. In line with government policy of the time, this established a system of competition between providers of nurse education to ensure value for money. Thus consortia of Regional Health Authorities came to purchase nurse education (and that of midwifery, health visiting and post-qualifying programmes) from universities (Francis and Humphreys, 1998). They were responsible for setting the conditions under which programmes of preparation for nurses operated, deciding the numbers of students that were required in order to meet the demands of workforce planning, and paying the universities for this activity. Consortia requirements were specified in contracts, which were monitored for issues of price, quality and attrition (drop-out rates), and they had the power to take qualifying and post-qualifying provision away from poorly performing providers. This meant that education providers had to respond to the local consortia requirements, which could take their business elsewhere (Quinn, 1995). These powers still apply today, although structures have altered since the 1990s.

Project 2000

Project 2000 had a major impact on nurse education. It introduced programmes of study with higher academic requirements in the late 1990s, to give students more opportunity to learn in practice without being used as 'pairs of hands'. In order to achieve this, nurse educators designed university programmes of study at diploma (equivalent to second-year degree) level, with a split of 50 per cent each for clinical practice and theory time in order to meet European Union Directives (those current in the 1990s were recently updated – see EUPC, 2005). Students were given 'super-numerary' status, so that they were no longer part of the established numbers on the wards. Local 'workforce development confederations' (WDCs), the new name for purchasing consortia, determined numbers of entrants. However, while attempting to address workforce planning needs, the NHS SHAs had planned based on NHS requirements alone, failing to realise that there were demands for nurses elsewhere, such as nursing homes, or that in the buoyant economic climate of the times there were other opportunities available in the job market. When WDCs reduced the numbers of pre-registration education places available, there were staff shortages throughout the NHS, at the same time as student nurses were less visible on the wards (Rivett, 2007).

Although a response to government demands, Project 2000 seems never to have been popular. It was criticised by government as being ineffective (DH, 1999b) as it was believed that supernumerary status reduced student nurses' clinical exposure, making them less able to work effectively at the point of initial registration (being not 'fit for practice'). In response to the changing nature of healthcare and in part to address newly qualified nurses' perceived skills shortages, the DH published its new nursing strategy, *Making a Difference* (1999b), which highlighted the contribution of nurses and their potential to improve their roles and responsibilities but was critical of nurses' more academic education.

The UKCC reviewed its strategy, publishing *Fitness for Practice* (UKCC, 1999). This concluded that nurses did indeed lack practical skills when they first qualified. As a result, Common Foundation Programmes (CFPs) were shortened from 18 months to one year, with earlier exposure to longer and more demanding clinical placements and to 24/7 shift patterns (Rivett, 2007). Nurse education programmes were restructured, and employers' and health authorities' concerns were addressed. University nursing departments undertook extensive consultation with local stake-holders when redesigning programmes, linking theoretical modules and practice outcomes to give a better indication of students' classroom learning and its relevance to the practice environment. Programmes are redesigned and undergo revalidation periodically to ensure that they are current and deliver qualified practitioners for changing healthcare needs.

In 2005, educational policy concerning fitness for practice at initial registration was reviewed (Moore, 2005), and UK issues were contrasted with those of other countries' regulatory bodies around the world. The report concluded that there was no evidence of 'policy failure', but that weaknesses in current arrangements should be addressed. These included pressure on clinical placements, which were having a negative impact on students' learning experiences (Hutchings et al., 2005); a shortage of clinical practice mentors and their inadequate role preparation; and the absence of valid, standard tools for assessing students in clinical practice placements (Moore, 2005).

The Nursing and Midwifery Council

The regulatory structure was again altered radically in 2002 when th
country's Boards for Nursing were replaced by the Nursing and M
(NMC), which is now the statutory body that regulates nursing and ensure
standards of education, training and professional practice are met. The NMC and
some of its recent policies are discussed in more detail in Chapter 7.

The influence of political parties, government health policy and Parliament

Throughout the preceding discussion, the role of government has been central to the
establishment of the registration of nurses, as the government was clearly concerned
that standards should be set for the profession, for training and for practitioners to
gain entry to the register.

UK health policy is a dynamic area. For some, the fact that the NHS is at the heart
of government means that it will always be closely contested at election times, and
will be the subject of continual change as political parties seek to stamp their mark on
it when elected. This means that change is a perpetual feature of UK health policy.
There are many influences on health policy changes, for example:

- political ideology;
- health policy specialists and advisers;
- pressure groups and the media;
- professionals and service providers;
- and, to an increasing extent, the views of patients, service users and their
carers.

Policy is also an adaptive process: if a change is made that does not work, it will be
reviewed and revised (Baggott, 2007).

Political parties

In the UK, two major political parties have formed governments in the post-WWII
period. These are the Conservative Party and the Labour Party. The UK political scene
is much more complicated than this, however, as there is a third major party, the
Liberal Democrats, and many smaller political parties, as well as independence
parties in Wales (Plaid Cymru) and in Scotland (the Scottish National Party). In
Northern Ireland, political debate includes the major UK parties but is also split
between republican parties (who want to join with the Irish Republic in the south of
the island, Eire) and unionists (who want to remain part of the UK). However, it is likely
that only Labour or Conservatives will form UK governments, so their political beliefs
are likely to continue to shape health policy.

Chapter 1 explored how the post-1979 Thatcher governments held different views
about the welfare state from those of previous ones. These changes were a result of
deep-seated ideological disagreements about the role of government and the state in

ple's lives. Although both parties agreed initially with the establishment of the NHS and its expansion, conflicts arose in the 1970s onwards because of the differing ideologies of the two parties, with Labour favouring collective approaches and the Conservatives favouring a greater role for individuals and families rather than the state. The Blair governments after 1997 (see Chapter 2) believed in and tried to implement a 'third way' approach, seeking to find a way distinct from these two pathways with, for the NHS, continued payment from taxation but devolution of authority from central government and a greater role for the private sector in service provision.

Activity 3.1

Political parties and health policy

In order better to understand the current health policies of Labour and the Conservatives, undertake the following activities.

Using the internet, find Labour's health policies online at www.labour.org.uk/ health. List what they believe are their chief achievements as a government. Then answer the following questions, based on your reading of the previous chapters in this book.

- Labour is proud that it has spent large sums of money on the health service.
  o Has this money made the system more efficient in terms of its productivity?
  o Has the employment situation become better or worse for nurses?
  o What do critics say about the constant reorganisations that the NHS has undergone since 1997?

Conservative pledges: autonomy and accountability

- Read the Conservatives' 2006 White Paper, *NHS Autonomy and Accountability*. It is available online at www.conservatives.com/ pdf/NHSautonomyandaccountability.pdf.

In a speech in 2007, Mark Simmonds (Conservative Shadow Health Minister; see www.conservatives.com/ and search under 'health') outlined Conservative ideas for the NHS as follows:

- The NHS is at the top of the Conservative's agenda and they will match the government's public spending figures.
- NHS problems are about more than just providing increased funds but are about their more efficient use. This government has constantly reorganised without investing in highly skilled staff to improve recovery and treatment rates.

The Department of Health

This is the principal government department with responsibility for UK health matters and for representing the country abroad, and it co-ordinates responses to threats such as infectious diseases. Other duties apply to England only (as Wales, Northern Ireland and Scotland Parliaments have taken on health policy responsibilities; see Chapter 2) and include:

- responsibilities for public health and the well-being of citizens;
- securing high quality services;
- promoting research.

The Secretary of State for Health is head politician for the NHS. He or she is appointed by the government in power, and is formally responsible to Parliament for what happens in the NHS. The Secretary of State leads legislation through Parliament, responds to questions and debates issues in Parliament, represents the NHS throughout government, and is assisted by ministers with various responsibilities and by permanent officials known as civil servants (Baggott, 2007), who are meant to give objective, non-political advice. Although a great deal of power still rests with the Secretary of State, in practice many powers have been devolved to lower levels, and both political parties are making noises about allowing this process to carry on so that service delivery is more responsive to local needs.

Additionally, within the system are the six Chief Officers. These are:

- Chief Medical Officer (CMO);
- Chief Dental Officer (CDO);
- Chief Pharmaceutical Officer (CPO);

- Chief Scientific Officer (CSO);
- Chief Allied Health Officer(CAHO);
- and for nursing, the Chief Nursing Officer (CNO).

The CNO has responsibility for delivering the government's strategy for nursing, and is the professional lead for all the nurses, midwives, health visitors and some professions allied to medicine in the NHS. The CNO publishes reports, guidance, advice and strategy, and these documents are available on the DH website.

Activity 3.2

In order better to understand the role of the Chief Nursing Officer and how her guidance has made an impact on nurses and nursing, undertake the following activities.

- *The NHS Plan* (2000) introduced the idea that nurses could begin to do more for patient care than they had previously. The CNO outlined ten key roles for nurses.
  - o Write down what you think these might be. Then, search the DH website (www.dh.gov.uk) for information about the CNO's ten key roles for nurses. Find the booklet *Developing Key Roles for Nurses and Midwives: A guide for managers* (DH, 2002), which gives some examples of how organisations have started to achieve these roles for practising nurses. Then find out what the ten key roles are and compare them with your own ideas.
  - o Next, read the examples from the booklet (DH, 2002) of how nurses have changed their roles.

- Search the DH website (www.dh.gov.uk) and find information about *Modernising Nursing Careers: Setting the direction* (DH, 2006d), which outlines directions in which career structures for qualified nurses should move in the future to respond to changes in the NHS and society.
  - o What does Christine Beasley as Chief Nursing Officer say that patients want from nurses?
  - o What are the four priority areas that *Modernising Nursing Careers* believes need addressing in order for change to be effective?

Some suggested answers are at the end of the chapter.

In addition to the role of political parties, civil servants and the professional leads, government health policy is also influenced in many ways depending on the views of individual MPs; special advisers to the government; influential clinicians and academics; pressure groups and lobbying organisations such as Age Concern or Mind (the National Association for Mental Health); and special advisers and external consultants.

Parliament

The government of the day is made up of representatives of the party that has won a General Election. The Queen, as Head of State, asks that party's leader to form a government. The party leader becomes the Prime Minister and invites chosen political figures to join the Cabinet. When the governing party has a large majority because of election success, it usually has the power to make sure that its policies and legislation pass easily through Parliament. It will have enough Members of Parliament (MPs) supporting its policy objectives to make sure that potential legislation (Bills) are not voted down in Parliament by the other parties and can become law (Acts of Parliament). Even so, Parliament will scrutinise potential legislation before it becomes law. MPs can ask questions in the House of Commons that ministers should answer, although they can refuse to do so. These debates can make good television viewing if there is a frank exchange of views, but they also have a serious side in that they allow difficult issues to be raised in a public forum, and can alert government to issues of concern in the country.

It is possible for backbenchers (those not in the government) to raise more formal Parliamentary debates, which may be reported in the media. Select Committees of the House of Commons are official investigations of policy, administration and financial issues. These give a level of detailed scrutiny to government actions and can be powerful bodies. They are meant to be non-partisan in the sense that they should contain MPs from all parties who should be impartial, but in reality Select Committees can be heavily influenced by party politics. There is a specific Health Policy Committee (Baggott, 2007).

MPs are allowed the opportunity to debate and discuss legislative proposals in Parliamentary debates as they pass through various stages and are drafted and redrafted. The House of Lords (the upper House of Parliament) also scrutinises Bills and makes recommendations at various stages. Even when a governing party has a large majority, Parliament can make them reconsider courses of action, hold up legislation and delay its enactment for long periods. In addition, individual citizens can appeal to their own MPs about personal matters, including health issues. Members of the public with serious complaints about the DH or the NHS can report these to the Health Ombudsman for England; similar roles exist in the other UK countries (Baggott, 2007). These are:

- the Scottish Public Services Ombudsman;
- the Northern Ireland Ombudsman;
- the Public Services Ombudsman for Wales.

The media's policy agenda influence

Over the last couple of decades the influence of the media in relation to health policy has grown and, as discussed later, arguably has played a central role in many recent policy developments. Baggott (2007) argues that health reporting is biased towards large hospital issues rather than community or public health issues, towards health 'scares' such as HIV/AIDS rather than issues of long-term care and chronic illness, and towards 'newsworthy stories', which may not reflect the general public's concerns.

The public perception of health can be created and distorted by media coverage. For example, the media has been accused of focusing on breast cancer as a risk for young women, covering stories where husbands and children have been left to carry on after the deaths of young women from the disease. These stories are sad and play with people's emotions, but in fact the greater risk for breast cancer lies with older women (Baggott, 2007) as 80 per cent of breast cancers are diagnosed in women of 50 and above (Cancer Research UK, 2008). How the media influences our perceptions of quality care issues is discussed further in Chapter 6.

When the media covers issues of rationing, health managers and NICE experts are portrayed as heartless bureaucrats when they rule that certain drug treatments should not be available, when actually these decisions are the result of complex economic calculations taking into account the cost of treatments compared to the benefits for individual patients and groups of patients in society. Nurses and doctors are portrayed as heroes in this, as they frequently speak up for patients based on their experiences of caring for small numbers of individuals rather than considering the bigger national picture of costs and benefits of treatments in a cash-limited service. One such example is the media presentation of issues surrounding treatment for Alzheimer's disease, which illustrates how a technical issue concerning costs and benefits of drug treatments can be presented in ways that the media define and control and are not necessarily factually accurate. For example, much television and news coverage took place when NICE recommended that drug treatments should no longer be available to those with mild Alzheimer's disease. *The Daily Telegraph* reported this in reasonable terms in several articles. Its Medical Editor (Hall, 2006) reported that the drugs cost about £900 per year, and 80,000 people would be affected by not being able to take them. Hall quoted Neil Hunt, of the Action on Alzheimer's Drugs Alliance, which represents charitable and professional organisations, as saying: *This is outrageous. It will rob families of precious time in the early stages of dementia and deprive people of comfort and dignity in the final stages of their lives.* Hall also quoted Professor Clive Ballard, a leading old-age psychiatrist, as saying: *Doctors will be forced into the impossible position of watching patients deteriorate before they prescribe drugs they know will help.* There were no counter-arguments from NICE in this piece to provide balance. In its prominent 'Comment' section, Jenny McCartney's (2006) headline was 'A Terrible Country in Which to Grow Old', and she argued that *Evidently politicians, like the rest of us, are simply shutting their eyes as their birthdays whirl around at horrifying speed, and praying it won't be them.*

Arguably, McCartney's views are a simplistic and distorted perspective of NICE's judgement. NICE produced a reasoned argument, taking into account the best evidence available. It recommended the drugs for use with moderate Alzheimer's disease rather than for every patient with a diagnosis (of whom there may be 290,000 in England and Wales according to NICE (2007)), and under the supervision of specialist clinicians with full assessment procedures and follow-up. The NICE committee considered a range of scientific evidence as well as the views of patients and carers, experts in the field, interest groups and pharmaceutical companies. They found that:

- the long-term evidence on the impact of these drug treatments on quality of life and on time to nursing home placement was limited and inconclusive;
- manufacturers' estimates as to the cost-effectiveness of the drugs were optimistic;
- there was no evidence to indicate positive benefits for carers.

Further research was recommended and the guidance is to be reviewed in 2009 (NICE, 2007). Therefore, arguably, this story was written as a news story in such a way as to offer some of the key features that Baggott (2007) identifies as important for newsworthiness. These are:

- some wider emotional appeal (it could be relevant to anybody);
- visual coverage of patients and carers (whose pictures were in the papers and on television);
- presentation in simple terms with victims (patients and carers), heroes (doctors and pressure group leaders) and villains (NICE 'bureaucrats');
- eye-catching headline potential.

Activity 3.3

In order better to understand how newsworthiness influences the reporting of health policy and practice issues in the newspapers and television, keep a log for a month on health-related stories you see and answer the following questions.

- How are the stories trying to draw your interest by manipulating your emotions?
- Are the victims, heroes and villains clearly identified and who are they?
- Is there balance in the sense that both (or more) sides are presented equally in any reports?
- Are the headlines eye-catching? Are they uplifting and positive or bleak and downcast?

As the answers will depend on the stories you encounter, there is no outline at the end of the chapter.

'Disasters', the media and health policy

Even if newsworthiness is a prime consideration in the media's reporting of health-related stories, 'disasters' are important areas for the media to cover, and the pressure that television and newspaper reporters exert on government can bring about real change. NHS disasters attract enormous media attention: in recent years, there have been many scandals leading to inquiries, such as:

- the Beverly Allitt Inquiry, instigated when a children's nurse became a serial killer of her patients;

- the Shipman Inquiry, when a GP was found guilty of murdering patients with opiates and became Britain's most prolific serial killer;
- the Alder Hey Hospital Inquiry, when staff at this Liverpool children's hospital were found guilty of poor and insensitive practice in relation to the removal, retention and disposal of human tissue and organs following post-mortems.

In 2007, the country was shocked by the media reporting of the failings of basic standards of care and management regarding the *clostridium difficile* outbreaks at Kent hospitals, and it is likely that criminal prosecutions may result from the Healthcare Commission report (see www.healthcarecommission.org.uk/home page.cfm).

However, in the late 1990s a series of dreadful events stood out, which were investigated by the Bristol Royal Infirmary Inquiry (BRII). This received extensive media coverage. Sandford (2003), for example, reporting for the British Broadcasting Corporation (BBC) listed a catalogue of recent health scandals, but remarked that the BRII was the most depressing, signalling *the moment when many people's trust in doctors first wavered significantly*. The government had to take action and introduced wide-ranging new areas of policy and legislation. The BRII final report (Kennedy, 2001) was published in 2001 but reviewed events in the paediatric heart surgery unit at the BRI between 1984 and 1995. Between these dates, paediatric surgeons at the BRI established a supra-regional centre for complex paediatric heart surgery, but the service was fatally flawed (Kennedy, 2001), with:

- no clear standards of care;
- inadequate resources, including too few appropriately qualified nurses;
- a lack of training or requirements for particular advanced skills for the senior surgeons involved;
- serious imbalances of power and a 'club culture', meaning that the views of the powerful medical elite were the only ones that counted;
- a failure to put the needs of sick children first.

These failings meant that, between 1991 and 1995, 30 or 35 more children under the age of one undergoing complex heart surgery died in the BRI than would have been expected in other units (Kennedy, 2001).

Unfortunately, there was no system of performance review and there were no standards of care, and surgeons were able to carry on operating when it was likely that they were exceeding their skill and knowledge. Unit staff raised concerns but no action was taken.

Major changes in the running of the NHS were already under way at the time; questions had been asked by the Thatcher government about the assumption that professionals, including doctors and nurses, should be allowed to continue with established systems of self-regulation; one of the functions of NHS general management was to manage healthcare professionals (HCPs) (see Chapter 1). However, one of the arguments doctors were able to use was that they were successful in regulating the profession through the Royal Colleges and the GMC. In the wake of the BRII, government was adamant that new systems of regulation and inspection would be put in place for all HCPs, and were able to use the BRII findings to support their determination. The list of BRII recommendations ran to 200; the DH has made much of its response, citing the BRII as a major driver in a large range of proposals to improve standards of care in the NHS (DH, 2006e). These are too numerous to list in full, but key features were:

- the strengthening of the work of NICE to publish guidance on standards of care, taking into account the public's and service users' views;
- post-1997, the Commission for Health Improvement (now the Healthcare Commission) and, latterly, Monitor were established as inspection bodies for NHS Trusts and Foundation Trusts respectively, including systems of clinical governance;
- the establishment of new agencies, the National Patient Safety Agency (NPSA), as a national system for reporting and analysing adverse events and 'near misses', and the National Clinical Assessment Authority (NCAA), a special health authority to support investigations of poor performance by doctors;
- National Service Frameworks (NSFs) to indicate national standards for a range of conditions (see Chapter 2).

Further information on all these areas can be obtained by searching the DH website (www.dh.gov.uk).

So, although the media may sometimes play a questionable role in health reporting, they can have a major influence on health policy and can help to bring about beneficial change through their reporting.

Trade unions, the Royal College of Nursing and the International Council of Nurses

The UK trade union movement has its roots in the socialist movements that featured in the Industrial Revolution, which was at its peak in the mid-nineteenth century. The influence of, and political pressure from, trade unions grew from around the beginning of the twentieth century. Trade unionism has always been strongly associated with the Labour Party and, indeed, trade unions are still a strong and influential voice within it. Many trade unions took a strongly socialist stance in the twentieth century, but their membership has fallen, as has their political militancy and their threat of strike action. Mrs Thatcher's government passed legislation limiting their powers, but trade unions still have an important role to play in safeguarding workers' rights, fighting for better pay and conditions, and securing more equal opportunities for women and ethnic minority people in the workplace. They also campaign and lobby MPs and government, including on health policy issues.

Nursing has not traditionally been a strongly unionised occupation. In the current NHS, the key trade union for nurses is Unison, which also represents NHS workers from other occupations, particularly domestic and portering staff. Trade unions and their umbrella organisation, the Trades Union Congress, have strong lobbying arms, which they use to try to influence health, employment and other government policies.

The Royal College of Nursing

From its establishment in 1916, the RCN has become the primary organisation representing the views of nurses at national and local level. It has about 300,000 UK members. However, it is neither a trade union like Unison, nor a regulatory body like the Royal Colleges of Physicians or Surgeons; it is the UK nurses' professional organisation. It is governed by a council, with representatives from all the UK's geographical areas and some student members. This council appoints a General Secretary, who is the head of the organisation. The RCN lists its mission statement on its website (www.rcn.org.uk) as being fivefold:

- to represent nurses' interests locally, nationally and internationally;
- to influence and lobby governments and others to implement policies that improve the quality of patient care and build on the importance to health outcomes of nurses, healthcare assistants and nursing students;
- to support and protect the value of nurses and nursing staff in all their diversity; their terms and conditions of employment; and their professional interests;
- to develop and educate nurses professionally and academically, building their resource of professional expertise and leadership; and of nursing's science, art of nursing and professional practice;
- to build a sustainable, member-led organisation capable of delivering its mission effectively, efficiently and in accordance with its values; and the systems, attitudes and resources to offer the best possible support and development to its staff.

In addition, the RCN provides professional and legal advice for individual nurses, responds to government policy initiatives on behalf of nurses, publishes its own guidance for nurses on a wide range of matters and supports networks of practice-related specialisms. It also lobbies politicians on health outcomes, and its annual conference always receives significant media attention, particularly when it is critical of the government of the day.

The International Council of Nurses

The International Council of Nurses (ICN) lists its mission statement on its website (www.icn.ch) as representing nursing worldwide, advancing the profession and influencing health policy. It is a federation of national nurses' associations from 128 countries. It was established in London in 1899 but is now based in Switzerland, and exists to ensure quality nursing care for all; good global health policies; and the advancement of a knowledgeable, professional, competent and satisfied nursing workforce.

The ICN has three goals and five core values. The three goals are:

- to bring nursing together worldwide;
- to advance nurses and nursing worldwide;
- to influence health policy.

The five core values are:

- visionary leadership;
- inclusiveness;
- flexibility;
- partnership;
- achievement.

The ICN produces a *Code of Ethics for Nurses* (ICN, 2006), which is an overarching statement of the principles and behaviours required for nurses globally to ensure that they meet ethical standards of practice and patient care. This sets out nurses' four fundamental responsibilities as being:

- the promotion of health;
- the prevention of illness;
- the restoration of health;
- the alleviation of suffering.

The ICN states:

The need for nursing is universal. Inherent in nursing is respect for human rights, including cultural rights, the right to life and choice, to dignity and to be treated with respect. Nursing care is respectful of and unrestricted by considerations of age, colour, creed, culture, disability or illness, gender, sexual orientation, nationality, politics, race or social status.

(2006, p3)

These principles are accepted across the world by the affiliated countries' nursing organisations, as are the ICN's standards and guidelines in other areas. The ICN is particularly active in professional nursing practice, nursing regulation and in regard to nurses' socio-economic welfare; it has formed a number of partnerships and strategic alliances with worldwide governmental and non-governmental agencies, foundations, regional groups, national associations and individuals.

CHAPTER SUMMARY

- Nurses have achieved registration as a result of exerting political pressure on government. Registration functions to protect the public by providing standards of entry and upholding standards of professional behaviour, and is a legal requirement for anyone seeking to work as a qualified nurse in the UK at Band 5 or above. Registration has undergone many changes in structure; the NMC is currently the UK body responsible for holding nurses' registrations.
- Politics will always influence how the NHS works and therefore the lives of the staff that work within it. There are many influences on governing political parties and many organisations seek to exert influence over them. Parliament is

the ultimate maker of laws, including those for health, and these laws are how health policies are enacted and turned into reality for the NHS and society.

- The media have a large role to play in shaping public and political attitudes towards health and health policy. However, a key criterion for them is that of newsworthiness, which can mean that reporting is not always completely accurate. The reporting of health 'disasters' can have a major impact on government, as evidenced by the policies of Blair governments and their regulatory frameworks for all HCPs, including nurses.
- The RCN is an important local and national 'voice' for nurses and nursing. The ICN is similarly influential internationally.
- These are important ideas for nurses to understand as they help directly to shape the scope of nursing care and the public's perception of nurses and nursing.

Activities: brief outline answers

3.1 Political parties and health policy (pages 46–7)

Labour's policies on health: chief achievements

- Since 1997 NHS spending has more than doubled, with over 32,000 more doctors and 85,000 more nurses.
- Largest ever NHS hospital building programme.
- Shorter waiting times; reduction in deaths from cancer, circulatory disease and coronary heart disease.
- Empowerment of patients through offering choice of at least four hospitals if further treatment is required.
- Helping people to lead healthier lives by taking prevention as seriously as cure; encouraging healthy living among the general public.

Some potential criticisms

Labour is proud that it has spent large sums of money on the health service.

- *Has this money made the system more efficient in terms of productivity?* Even the objective analysis of Wanless et al. (2007) found that there was at present no firm evidence that this extra spending had produced substantial benefits.
- *Has the employment situation become better or worse for nurses?* In 2007, many nurses leaving training were unable to secure jobs on registration, some long-qualified nurses failed to secure jobs as their posts were reviewed under Agenda for Change job evaluation, and training places were cut back in university departments as the financial crisis hit.
- *What do critics say about the constant reorganisations that the NHS has undergone since 1997?* That these have been costly and a waste of money (Toynbee, 2007).

Conservative pledges: autonomy and accountability

- *If Conservatives will reduce central government interference, what will be the role of government?* They outline a strategy in which central government will oversee the work of the NHS Board, which will report to them on their activities.

- *What would be the benefits of an NHS Board?* It would, in theory, be the independent management body for the NHS and would stop politicians manipulating and changing NHS priorities for their own ends, particularly around election times, and allow a focus on outcomes in terms of treatment successes rather than government targets.
- *As a future qualified nurse, what do this White Paper's proposals offer you?* Little is aimed at nurses, but the proposals talk about greater autonomy for professionals in workforce planning, education and training, and career pathways.

3.2 The Chief Nursing Officer and Modernising Nursing Careers (page 48)

The ten key roles outlined by the CNO are:

- To order diagnostic investigations such as pathology tests and X-rays.
- To make and receive referrals direct, say, to a therapist or pain consultant.
- To admit and discharge patients for specified conditions and within agreed protocols.
- To manage patient caseloads, say, for diabetes or rheumatology.
- To run clinics, say, for ophthalmology or dermatology.
- To prescribe medicines and treatments.
- To carry out a wide range of resuscitation procedures, including defibrillation.
- To perform minor surgery and outpatient procedures.
- To triage patients using the latest information technology to the most appropriate health professional.
- To take a lead in the way local health services are organised and in the way that they are run.

- The examples of how nurses have changed their roles from the booklet, *Modernising Nursing Careers: Setting the direction* (DH, 2006d) will be relevant to you in your placement areas because you will see nurses performing them and when you qualify because you will be expected to undertake them.

- *What does Christine Beasley as Chief Nursing Officer say that patients want from nurses?* She says:

In spite of all this change, what patients want and need from nurses has changed very little. Patients want their contact with nurses to make them feel safe, cared for, respected and involved. They want to know that the nurse is there unconditionally for them, especially when faced with fear, pain or loss. They want to know that nurses' actions will be in their best interests and will help them get better, keep well, live life to the full, or help towards a better death. This may sound obvious, almost simple, after all it is what nursing is and has always been about.

(DH, 2006d, p6)

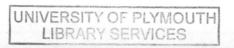

- *What are the four priority areas that* Modernising Nursing Careers *believes should be addressed for change to be effective?* They are (DH, 2006d, p19):
  o   Develop a competent and flexible nursing workforce.
  o   Update career pathways and career choices.
  o   Prepare nurses to lead in a changed healthcare system.
  o   Modernise the image of nursing and nursing careers.

Knowledge review

Having completed the chapter, how would you now rate your knowledge of the following topics?

	Good	Adequate	Poor
1. How the registration of nursing evolved.			
2. How nurse education has developed recently.			
3. The roles of political parties, government and Parliament in shaping health policies.			
4. The role of the Chief Nursing Officer.			
5. How the press and television present health policy topics and influence the policy agenda.			
6. The roles of trade unions, the Royal College of Nursing (RCN) and the International Council of Nurses (ICN).			

Further reading

Abel-Smith, B (1960) *A History of the Nursing Profession.* London: Heinemann.

Baggott, R (2007) *Understanding Health Policy.* Bristol: The Policy Press.

Hart, C (2004) *Nurses and Politics: The impact of power and practice.* Basingstoke: Palgrave Macmillan.

Rafferty, AM (1996) *The Politics of Nursing Knowledge.* London: Routledge.

Useful websites

www.icn.ch/ International Council of Nurses (ICN) website.

www.labour-party.org.uk/manifestos/ Labour Party manifestos (where they set out their policies if elected) for 1997 and 2001.

www.nhshistory.com NHS history site, run by Geoffrey Rivett.

www.nmc-uk.org/ The official website of the Nursing and Midwifery Council – the governing body for nurses and midwives.

www.opsi.gov.uk/si/si2002/20020253.htm#3 For the full text of the statutory order creating the NMC.

www.rcn.org.uk Royal College of Nursing (RCN): the professional association for nurses. Similar in some respects to a trade union.

Chapter 4

The caring culture and tradition in nursing

NMC Standards of Proficiency

This chapter will address the following NMC *Standards of Proficiency* and *Outcomes to be achieved for entry to the branch programme.*

Practise in a fair and anti-discriminatory way, acknowledging the differences in beliefs and cultural practices of individuals or groups.

Outcomes to be achieved for entry to the branch programme:
Demonstrate the importance of promoting equity in patient and client care by contributing to nursing care in a fair and anti-discriminatory way:

- demonstrate fairness and sensitivity when responding to patients, clients and groups from diverse circumstances;
- recognise the needs of patients and clients whose lives are affected by disability, however manifest.

Engage in, develop and disengage from therapeutic relationships through the use of appropriate communication and interpersonal skills.

Outcomes to be achieved for entry to the branch programme:
Discuss methods of, barriers to, and the boundaries of, effective communication and interpersonal relationships:

- recognise the effect of one's own values on interactions with patients and clients and their carers, families and friends;
- utilise appropriate communication skills with patients and clients;
- acknowledge the boundaries of a professional caring relationship.

Demonstrate sensitivity when interacting with and providing information to patients and clients.

Provide a rationale for the nursing care delivered which takes account of social, cultural, spiritual, legal, political and economic influences.

Chapter aims

After reading this chapter, you will able to outline:

- an understanding of the caring culture and tradition in nursing, including the impact of Florence Nightingale and Mary Seacole;
- an appreciation of how issues of gender can influence caring;
- an understanding of the distinction between 'caring for' and 'caring about';
- an overview of caring in a diverse and multicultural context.

Introduction

In this chapter we will examine ideas about the caring tradition in nursing, including the impact of Florence Nightingale and Mary Seacole, the distinction between 'caring for' and 'caring about', issues of gender, and caring in a diverse and multicultural context.

Despite the picture of organisational change presented in Chapters 1 and 2, it is important to remember that treatment and care continue, provided by HCPs whose job it is to look after sick and needy people regardless of the NHS reorganisation currently under way. This human caring is perhaps the one unchanging, constant factor that has been operating since time began; despite the fact that, in the UK, we have chosen to organise our healthcare services in a particular fashion, sick and needy people require care from others and will continue to do so whatever form of health service is in existence.

In this chapter we will be looking at concepts of caring. We will begin with a brief mention of the impact of key figures in the history of nursing, Florence Nightingale and Mary Seacole. They lived in a very different society from our own, and so we will examine some more contemporary ideas about what caring is and how it is affected by gender issues, and finally the impact that multiculturalism is having on caring in today's health service.

Florence Nightingale

Florence Nightingale (1820–1910) was a remarkable woman, in the sense that she overcame many personal and social obstacles to become influential in her time. She was born a second daughter to a wealthy family in a society with rigid class divisions and very fixed views on the role of women; she was lucky that her father was an educated man and was keen to make sure that his daughters received schooling, because at that time it was considered unnecessary to educate women, whose lives were likely to be spent in homemaking and childcare. However, it seems that Nightingale was convinced from an early age that she had as her destiny some special purpose or role in society. She was chronically shy and ill at ease with others as a child, and found her early years difficult if not boring, but in early adulthood she became a beautiful and accomplished socialite and also developed deeply held religious convictions (Holliday and Parker, 1997). She decided on nursing as an outlet for her talents, but faced much hostility and was denied this opportunity by her parents, who viewed this as an entirely unsuitable occupation for a woman from the upper classes: nurses at that time were generally low-class women not known for their professionalism, compassion or sobriety.

Nightingale eventually broke with her family and trained for three months in Kaiserworth in Germany under the auspices of a religious order in which deaconesses cared for the sick, eventually returning home in 1853 to become superintendent of a small hospital called the Establishment for Gentlewomen During Illness at No. 1 Harley Street, London. Here she put into practice what she had learned. She believed in the 'miasma' theory of disease causation, meaning that noxious odours circulating in the atmosphere were responsible for ill health. Although this theory was disproved when the role of germs in illness was discovered, Nightingale refused to understand these ideas but still managed to be effective through rudimentary public health measures of hygiene and fresh air (Basford, 1995). However, it was her work with soldiers of the British Army in the Crimean War that established her fame.

Nightingale arrived in Scutari, Turkey, in 1854, and found that Army casualties were dying of neglect as little or no provision was made for them. Consequently, as well as their battlefield injuries, the soldiers had to cope with malnutrition, and unsanitary water supplies and facilities, and diseases such as dysentery and cholera were rife. Having been appointed by her friend Sydney Herbert, an important government figure, she had the authority to begin reform, and despite opposition from the military establishment she and her team began to secure access to good-quality supplies of food and water, and to establish basic standards of cleanliness and hygiene in the wards where soldiers were looked after (Basford, 1995). She also played a role in personally caring for the soldiers, writing letters to their families and befriending them, and came to be revered as a ministering heroine and portrayed at home as the angelic 'lady with the lamp'. Although she probably disliked the publicity, it is clear that this positive image helped her in her demands for supplies and increased her status in the Crimea. In Scutari she developed her ideas concerning the need for nurse training so that nursing could take its place as the servant of medicine, rather than nurses serving doctors, laying the foundations for a professional status for nurses that were only fully built over a century later (Holliday and Parker, 1997).

Returning from the Crimean War in 1856, Nightingale hid herself away from the public gaze but continued working on the reform of hospital services. In 1860 she founded the Nightingale School of Nursing at St Thomas's Hospital in London with money collected from public subscriptions in recognition of her work in the Crimea. Her approach was that nurses needed appropriate training for their roles, and so her Probationer nurses received a year's training, mostly in supervised practical work under a hospital ward sister. 'Her' nurses went on to found similar training establishments in this country and abroad. In this way Nightingale contributed directly to standards of care as well as to improving the status of nurses and nursing through her public popularity, organisational skills and insistence on hygiene and good public health measures (Florence Nightingale Museum Trust, 2003). She was one of nursing's first great leaders.

Mary Seacole

Mary Seacole's story is very different from that of Florence Nightingale, but she demonstrated leadership, fortitude and heroism in no small measure. She was a contemporary of Nightingale who also cared for soldiers in the Crimean War and became familiar and respected in Victorian society, but whose name and achievements are now much less celebrated.

Born in Jamaica in 1805, Seacole learned her skills from her mother, who was a 'healer' in her society and used a range of traditional Creole remedies in ministering to the sick (Stuart, undated) – talents that were put to good use as Seacole earned her living from them. She married an English sailor, Edwin Seacole, godson of Lord Nelson, but when he died young she required an outlet for her talents and, as a restless soul, decided to go to the Crimea to help the wounded. She initially went to England and volunteered her services to Nightingale's organisation and to the War Office, but was rejected, probably because of her colour and because she not of the class or background that was acceptable to Nightingale, who was not keen on Seacole personally (Stuart, undated). Instead, she went to the Crimea at her own expense and established a servicemen's hostel known as the British Hostel (Anionwu, 2006), the profits from which financed her other war activities. Rather than establishing a hospital network in parallel to that of Nightingale, Seacole tended to battlefield casualties, many with horrific injuries, under fire of guns and in almost constant danger, treating wounds with the traditional remedies that she had learnt at home in the West Indies.

Seacole was destitute when the war finished and returned to London in dire straits. However, as her activities had been reported widely in England, she too had a reputation as a national heroine, being known as 'Mother' or 'Aunty' to the soldiers for whom she cared (Stuart, undated). A public subscription was raised that saved her, and her autobiography (published in 1857) was a best-seller. In its preface, the contemporary newspaper reporter WH Russell (1857) describes her thus:

> I have witnessed her devotion and her courage; I have already borne testimony to her services to all who needed them. She is the first who has redeemed the name of 'sutler' [a battlefield follower] from the suspicion of worthlessness, mercenary baseness, and plunder; and I trust that England will not forget one who nursed her sick, who sought out her wounded to aid and succour them, and who performed the last offices for some of her illustrious dead.

She became a popular figure in Victorian society, a larger-than-life person, and friendly with the Royal Family. She died in 1881, alas without establishing a rapport with Nightingale, but her legacy is one of personal courage in the face of racism and of dangerous conditions. British Army medical personnel were frequently dismissive of the skills that her patients valued so highly (Stuart, undated); but, like Nightingale, she demonstrated that nurses could make an effective contribution to treatment and care of the sick, independent from that of medicine.

In order to begin to understand the obstacles and prejudices that these two women faced, and to reflect on their achievement, work through the following exercises.

- The activities of Florence Nightingale and Mary Seacole were shaped by the society in which they lived.
    - What was the Victorian attitude towards women and how did they view their status and responsibilities?
    - What was the popular image of nurses and nursing at the time?

A brief outline of what you might find is at the end of the chapter.

Caring in healthcare

Caring is identified as a difficult concept to define (Bassett, 2002; van Hooft, 2006), but is still held as being utterly central to understanding what nurses do, as well as being attributable in some measure to all human societies (Kyle, 1995). Much discussion in the literature concerns aspects of care from philosophical, ethical and spiritual perspectives (Kyle, 1995; van Hooft, 2006), although Paley (2001) argues that, despite numerous volumes and much research being written on the subject, there is no clear definition of what constitutes caring because attempting to pin it down is in itself an impossible task.

For some, there is a distinction to be drawn between 'caring for' and 'caring about', in the sense that 'caring for' means the process of caregiving, while 'caring about' means having an emotional connection with another person, wishing them well and acting in their best interests (Davies, 1995). In nursing, these factors are combined so that the relationship between a nurse and a patient, for example, is characterised by the practicalities of giving technically proficient and professionally bounded care, but is also dependent on the establishment and maintenance of an interpersonal relationship (Liu et al., 2006; van Hooft, 2006). This is quite different from other occupations and professions, and sets nurses aside in the depth and meaning of their relationships with their clients. A 'desire' or 'need' to care is also discussed as the 'calling' that brings nurses into their professions, and the values they find provide an enduring sense of purpose; a timeless ethic, but one that is often threatened by the production-line processes (Watson, 2006) in modern healthcare, including the NHS.

Many in healthcare go into the various professions in order to care for others, to 'make a difference' and because they know that a unique sense of personal and professional satisfaction ensues when one gives of oneself to others. For some this can be a function of personal religious beliefs; for others it is a manifestation of more human attributes such as altruism. We will all need care at some point in our lives, and at some level most people are capable of caring for others.

It is clear from the literature that 'caring' is conceptualised as an elemental human property, and one requires some degree of 'trusting', 'sharing' and 'openness' to the needs of others. This is an essential feature of nursing as it is 'privileged' by the intimate relationships that nurses have with those in their care, and good communication skills and the ability to offer empathy and compassion are necessary in order for caring to be effective (van Hooft, 2006). Caring, and thus nursing, is much more than the exercise of certain skills or competencies in a professional manner, even if professional, legal and organisational requirements underpin relationships between nurses and clients:

> The mere exercise of caring behaviours without regard to the spirit that these activities are engaged in is not adequate. Therapeutically necessary levels of trust and communication with clients are not likely to be set up by nurses who are no more than coldly efficient in the exercise of their professional duties.
>
> (van Hooft, 2006, p11)

Van Hooft (2006) uses the term 'professional commitment', meaning that a nurse takes a stance towards a specific person and their health and well-being for a period of time – a similar concept to 'obligation' in that it indicates what the nurse 'ought' to say and do, and this will reflect training, education and socialisation in the chosen role. So, a professionally committed nurse cares about the healthcare needs of clients and thus responds to the needs shown in their assessment, and identified as a result of professional education and experience. As 'health' is a vague term, caring for a patient's healthcare needs will depend on individual and societal norms and values.

Gender issues in healthcare

In Chapter 1 you read a quote about the role of nurses through the eyes of a St George's Hospital Probationer and were asked to consider how the image of women in society has changed, and how nurses are perceived in healthcare today. Above, we saw how Mary Seacole and Florence Nightingale took on 'caring' roles in disobedience of the prevailing norms of the society in which they lived, but the norms they transgressed were concerned with race and class, not gender, because in their society as well as in ours today the prevailing image of someone who 'cares' is that of a female. In this section we are going to look at some ideas about how gender affects the roles that women tend to play and hence how caring occupations are 'gendered'.

Caring and emotional labour

If healthcare work requires 'caring' and an emotional connection, in our society this is widely still perceived as 'women's work', and these types of connections are long-established and remain pervasive (van Hooft, 2006). Women are seen as emotional and able to cope with the emotions of others, just as women are held to do in the family with husbands and children, and these emotional aspects of caring work are also central to the work and the purpose of healthcare (Staden, 1998). These issues are also largely 'invisible' – they cannot be costed and, until comparatively recently, they have not been measurable in any sense (Watson, 2002), but, even so, they remain the essence and uniqueness of nursing (Bassett, 2002), and are an intimate and powerful connection between practitioners and their clients.

Nurses are the 'front line', closest to patients and in contact with them for 24 hours a day. They also see people at their most vulnerable and most needy, and are required to respond to such emotional states – an example of an occupation that uses 'emotional labour' (Bolton, 2000). Such caring activity is about action and reaction, doing and being, and involves responses to another person's needs and an exchange between patient and nurse.

Research summary

Emotional labour

'Emotional labour' in nursing and the caring professions is a term now generally accepted and in common currency, and there is a growing body of theoretical and empirical literature on the issue. Hunter (2001) reviewed the literature on emotional work, using an extensive search of midwifery, nursing and social science sources to inform her ideas. She highlights the contribution of Hochschild, whose 1983 publication, *The Managed Heart: Commercialization of human feeling*, was the first scholarly work to identify 'emotional labour' as:

> when people use their personal interactions to create positive moods and feelings in others. This is more than simple acting and also requires the creation of these feelings in themselves.

As Hochschild puts it, *the emotional style of offering the service is part of the service itself* (2003, p5).

Hunter (2001) quotes several sources of critical literature, making the point that Hochschild's work was based on US flight attendants, may not transfer directly to the UK NHS and that emotional labour may be much more complex than Hochschild suggests.

However, consensus exists that emotional labour:

- is essential for good nursing care;
- is not without cost to the worker (Phillips, 1996);
- may cause occupational stress and burnout from the constant need for nurses to manage the emotions of others (McVicar, 2003);
- is largely invisible but requires a high level of skills among practitioners (Staden, 1998);
- is seen as a 'natural female skill' and is also often in evidence in managing inter-professional relationships between doctors and nurses (Timmons and Tanner, 2005) as well as with patients and clients.

Bolton (2000) argues that emotional labour is more than simply acting, entailing genuine and authentic interaction between staff and clients, and that this authentic emotional work should be seen as a 'gift' from nurse to patient.

Caring and gender inequalities

We also noted in Chapter 1 that doctors have traditionally had power in healthcare organisations and this stems from their position in society as key decision makers. A society dominated by men is known as a patriarchal society. Sociologists argue that this type of social organisation has consequences for men and women – essentially that men's powerful social and economic positions mean that in any exchange or interaction, women's positions are less powerful, so a patriarchal society is one in which women are disadvantaged because of their gender (Bradley, 1994). This goes back centuries, so:

> Men have been kings, writers, composers, thinkers and doers, women have been wives, mistresses, friends, and helpmates. The very word woman, in fact, emphasises this dependent anonymous position. It derives from the Anglo Saxon wifman, literally 'wife-man'.
>
> (Bullough, 1974, quoted in Oakley, 1981, p69)

The Functionalist sociologist Talcott Parsons (1956) argued that, in the twentieth-century USA, the successful society in which he lived, for society to continue to function, women were required to have 'expressive' roles, such as nurturing, caring and childcare, and their activities were thus confined to the home and family. He saw men's roles as being 'instrumental', making things happen and taking the lead in all situations, and they thus operated within the family as well as the wider society.

For feminists such as Oakley (1981), this 'traditional' image of the role of women is prejudicial, discriminatory and simply wrong, having four elements that affect how men see women and how women see themselves. Therefore, patriarchal ideas in society condemn women to passivity, instability, materiality and maternalism. For van Hooft (2006), female thinking about personal health, for example, emphasises traditional concepts of fecundity and nurturing, and is very different from masculine ones of 'soldiering on' and providing for a family.

Thus, as the roles played by men and women in society are deeply ingrained, these modes of thinking and behaviour have a large effect on their roles within healthcare settings; public perceptions of women and of nursing mean that a good nurse = a good woman, and nursing is thus a fundamentally gendered occupation. Arguably, society sees nursing as 'women's work'; this is understandable considering that women's work within society has always been substantially about caring and nurturing. Even today, nursing is still made up of only approximately 10 per cent men (Buchan and Seccombe, 2004); these small numbers are reflected in the fact that a male nurse will still be called a 'male nurse', while the term 'nurse' always relates to a female in the eyes of the general public. So, this image of women as carers is 'socially constructed', meaning that it is produced by people within society, and it influences how women see themselves as people and as carers. As doctors and medicine are more powerful within society and the NHS than women and nurses, healthcare is another area where inequality exists for women (Davies, 1995).

Activity 4.2

In order to begin to understand how gender inequalities occur within health-care and the many forms of potential disadvantage that are in evidence, read the examples below and undertake the activities by personal observation, talking to colleagues and internet searches.

- Healthcare roles other than medicine are still viewed by society as mundane ('caring' rather than 'curing'; 'looking after' rather than 'treating') and as women's work; women do them because it is 'natural' for them to do so.
  - Find out what the terms 'vocation' and 'profession' mean. Is nursing a vocation or a profession?
- The pay and status of nursing are less than that of medicine. For example, at the top of their salary scales after eight years in post, in 2007, the annual salary of a Nurse Consultant (Band 8c) was approximately £61,000, while that of a Hospital medical or surgical Consultant was approximately £96,000 and with excellence awards and private practice the sum for most medical Consultants reached well over £100,000.
  - Compare the roles of Nurse Consultants to those of Hospital medical or surgical ones. What is it about their roles and responsibilities that means doctors earn more than nurses?

A brief outline of what you might find is at the end of the chapter.

The 'hidden voice of nursing'?

The *hidden voice of nursing* (Davies, 1995) is a concept that reflects how nursing can be argued to lack power and identity because it is a female gendered occupation (Benner and Wrubel, 1989), but it is not a straightforward concept.

Nurses are frequently concerned with 'getting the work done', or achieving beneficial outcomes for patients whatever is required, and a great deal of nursing work is about problem solving, risk avoidance and making sure that the contributions of other professions are successfully integrated into patient care management. However, there is more to this than meets the eye (Davies, 1995): Stein's (1967) classic study illustrated how nurses made suggestions and 'steered' doctors towards decisions that were the appropriate courses of action by tact rather than conflict and that these forms of interaction were largely dependent on gender: a 'doctor–nurse game' was played out in all healthcare settings (Stein, 1967). When these ideas were revisited (Stein et al., 1990), the issues were not so obvious as there was less subtle steering and more assertiveness on show among the nurses; the increasing number of female doctors and changes within the wider society have also changed the highly patri-archical relationships (Porter, 1992) seen by Stein in the 1960s (Davies, 1995).

Activity 4.3

In order to begin to understand how experienced nurses overcome power and gender inequalities in the best interests of their patients, work through the following activities.

- Observe the interactions between doctors and nurses during several shifts.
  - ○ How is it that nurses make their voices heard as patient advocates?
- Experienced nurses are very skilled at achieving successful outcomes for patients, but what works best in what circumstances? Note the circumstances where nurses may be passive, assertive and aggressive in their dealings with doctors.
  - ○ Which was the most successful approach and why?

The answers to these questions will be dependent on what you see happening locally, so there is no outline at the end of the chapter.

Inequality of opportunity in the NHS

As well as the sociological explanations discussed above, Adams (1994) identified three other factors predisposing women to inequality of opportunity within the NHS itself.

- Trade-off between family and career: once a break has been taken, it is very difficult to 'pick up the threads' again.
- Approximately a third of women in the NHS worked part-time in 1994, which may give disadvantage in terms of further education and training, or promotions, as the organisation is not flexible enough to allow this.
- Uniformly poor childcare provision in terms of cost, availability and opening hours. NHS provision for staff is often not available at times convenient for nursing shifts, or there are not enough places for all staff who want them, and it is frequently difficult to arrange other paid childcare around shift patterns.

Despite initiatives to overcome these problems, there has been limited success in overturning them (Adams 1994; Corby 1995), but recent legislation in the form of the Work and Families Act 2006 seeks to make a difference to women's opportunities within the NHS in relation to maternity provision. NHS organisations are now required to have appropriate strategies in place by April 2007 for gender equality, particularly in regard to pay (NHS Employers, 2007), in recognition of the limited success of the 1975 Sex Discrimination Act in this area (for further information about the 2006 Act consult the Office for Public Sector Information at www.opsi.gov.uk/).

Caring in a diverse and multicultural context

In the past 50 years the cultural make-up of the UK has changed. As indicated by the research summary below, net migration of people to these islands has meant that people from many different cultures now live in the UK. These people require health services, and their religious beliefs and social attitudes mean that caring for them may not be the same as caring for people from the same culture as oneself, and, indeed, that some of our underlying beliefs and attitudes are actually offensive to these incomers in some way. This section is intended to give an overview of the issues involved in caring for people from other cultures, although it is not possible to give a guide to exactly how people from different religious and cultural traditions need to be looked after and for this it may be necessary to contact local religious practitioners from faiths concerned (hospital switchboards should have contact telephone numbers).

Research summary

Population growth and migration

By mid-2005 the UK had a population of 60.2 million people (50.4 million in England), and this population is growing, by 375,100 people in the year to mid-2005 (0.6 per cent), and by 7.7 per cent since 1971 (from 55.9 million). Growth has accelerated in recent years due to mass immigration, although birth rates are falling. The population is also an ageing one, with an average age of 38 years and one in six of the population aged over 65 years (National Statistics Population Trends, 2006).

Figure 4.1 shows how the population growth was made up between 1993 and 2002: more people are coming to the UK to live here than are leaving to live abroad.

For England and Wales, migration in 2004 totalled 217,000 people: 542,000 in-migrants and 325,000 out-migrants. Between 1995 and 2004, inflows and outflows have been increasing steadily with a sharp increase in inflows in 2004, mainly due to increased freedom of movement within the European Union (EU)

Figure 4.1: International migration from and to the UK.

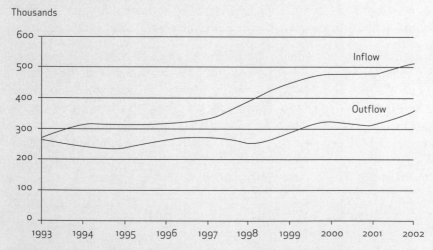

Source: From National Statistics online: *People and Migration* (December 2005), National Statistics website: www.statistics.gov.uk. Crown copyright material is reproduced with the permission of the Controller of HMSO. Reproduced under the terms of the Click-Use Licence.

for citizens from Central and Eastern European countries since their accession to the EU in May 2004. Most migrants chose to live in the southeast of England (National Statistics Population Trends, 2006).

Table 4.1 shows the population of the UK by ethnic group and indicates that, in 2001, 7.9 per cent of the population were from ethnic origins other than 'white', of which approximately 50 per cent were of Asian descent and 25 per cent Black. These figures indicate that the UK is a culturally diverse or 'multicultural' nation in the twenty-first century.

Table 4.1:   Population of the UK by ethnic group, April 2001.

Ethnic group	Total population		Non-white population
	(Numbers)	(Percentages)	(Percentages)
White	54,153,898	92.1	–
Mixed	677,117	1.2	14.6
Indian	1,053,411	1.8	22.7
Pakistani	747,285	1.3	16.1
Bangladeshi	283,063	0.5	6.1
Other Asian	247,664	0.4	5.3
All Asian or Asian British	2,331,423	4.0	50.3
Black Caribbean	565,876	1.0	12.2
Black African	485,277	0.8	10.5
Black Other	97,585	0.2	2.1
All Black or Black British	1,148,738	2.0	24.8
Chinese	247,403	0.4	5.3
Other ethnic groups	230,615	0.4	5.0
All minority ethnic population	4,635,296	7.9	100.0
All population	58,789,194	100.0	

Source: From National Statistics online: *People and Migration* (December 2005), National Statistics website: www.statistics.gov.uk. Crown copyright material is reproduced with the permission of the Controller of HMSO. Reproduced under the terms of the Click-Use Licence.

Multiculturalism and health

The UK has been thriving economically for many years and the majority of immigrants arrive to take advantage of this and to provide a better life for themselves and their families, although in recent times there has also been a trend for people seeking asylum here from dangerous circumstances in their own countries.

Whatever the reason for moving to the UK, it is important to remember that people arriving here may be very proud of their own cultural heritage and be reluctant to change their language, religion, eating habits and ways of behaviour. These provide a sense of self and identity for themselves as individuals and for their community in a new and unfamiliar world (Johnson, 2003). Even people who are willing to assimilate completely will take time to do so. As there is no legal requirement that migrants should make such changes, only the broad need to adhere to the laws of the land, the UK will continue to be a society that welcomes those from very different back-grounds. Diverse communities will continue to flourish, particularly in inner-city areas, towards which new arrivals tend to gravitate; for example, half the UK population of Bangladeshis live in the East End of London, and over 300 languages are estimated to be spoken in London (Johnson, 2003).

Although economic activity and achievement patterns are complex and changing over time, generally speaking, sources of disadvantage for many new arrivals and for those in established communities are poverty and unemployment, inadequate spoken and written English, intolerant attitudes and racism from host communities, and poorer health status. However, it is important not to generalise and assume that *all* migrants have poorer health in all conditions, as disease rates for the major hospital admissions and killers vary by ethnic origin (Kai and Bhopal, 2003): a good summary of these differences and other issues to do with illness and treatment is found in Kai (2003, Chapter 2).

One area of inequality that has received a lot of attention recently is ethnic minority care in mental health, largely because mental health diagnoses are highly dependent on context; they relate to transgressing the 'normal' in some way, and normal is defined by the society in which this transgression takes place (Patel, 2003).

Many religious traditions are represented among migrants, with substantial populations of Muslims, Hindus and Sikhs now worshipping here alongside Christians and Jews. These people all have different spiritual needs and require cultural sensitivity from nurses and, while it is not the attempt of this section to outline these needs, you should be familiar with the services and support provided by your local Trust, which is likely to have links with local community and religious groups offering care, support and guidance.

Transcultural nursing

The kinds of inequalities outlined above can have a profound impact on the quality of care received. In a health service that aspires to provide equality of access and treatment for all regardless of race or culture, it is important for nurses to do everything they can to ensure a high quality of care and service for all. This has led to the establishment of transcultural health and social care as a field of study, examining comparative patterns of health and illness and their relationship to culture, as well as issues surrounding the provision of care that is competent to meet the needs of people in cultures other than ours, and is sensitive in doing so (Papadopoulos, 2006). Thus there is a commitment to anti-oppressive and anti-discriminatory practice, and to examining how organisations and societies may, however unwittingly, create and maintain disadvantage. These values are reflected in the educational requirements of the *NMC Code of Professional Conduct* (2008) and the Quality Assurance Agency (QAA, 2001), as well as in a legal requirement that organisations train staff to address the needs of other cultures (Race Relations (amendment) Act 2000).

Cultural competence (Papadopoulos, 2006) is a term that indicates the capacity to provide effective care and takes into account others' cultural beliefs and preferences. The underpinning values emphasise:

- the individual, each of whom has inherent worth;
- culture, which we all have and which influences our behaviour and beliefs;
- structure, whose power can be enabling or disabling;
- health and illness, states of which are culturally defined;
- caring, which responds to the uniqueness of the individual in a culturally sensitive manner;
- nursing, whose activity should be culturally competent;
- cultural competence, a process for continuously developing and refining one's capacity for effective healthcare, which responds to cultural factors.

Papadopoulos et al. formulated a model for developing cultural competence (Papadopoulos, 2006; see Figure 4.2). Its four elements require us to examine our

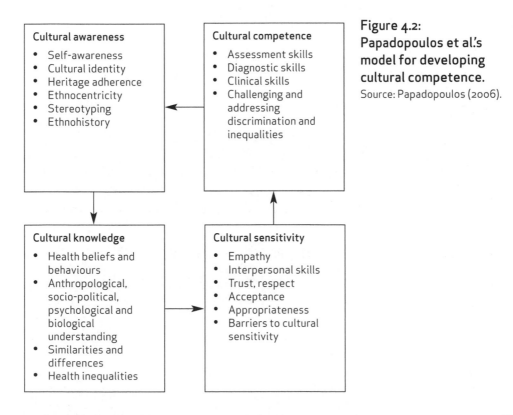

Figure 4.2:
Papadopoulos et al.'s model for developing cultural competence.
Source: Papadopoulos (2006).

own values and beliefs, attempting to provide culturally appropriate care, but also addressing wider issues such as inequalities in society. Once cultural awareness, knowledge and sensitivity are attained, it should be possible to give culturally competent care to those from other cultures and, although it will be impossible to have a working knowledge of all cultures, it should be possible to acquire the requisite understanding of new cultures encountered. In this way nurses can move along a continuum from:

1. culturally incompetent practice, to
2. culturally aware practice, to
3. culturally safe practice, to
4. culturally competent practice.

UK legislation and the NHS

Although there has been much legislation promoting race equality and race relations since the 1960s, it was not until the Race Relations (amendment) Act (2000) that the NHS has been required to protect individuals and groups from racial discrimination and to promote racial equality in the workplace. UK institutions have been explicitly criticised in enquiries such as that of McPherson et al. (1999), which labelled the Metropolitan Police institutionally racist following their mishandling of the Stephen Lawrence murder case. Institutional racism means the failure to provide an acceptable service because of race or colour. Thus NHS Trusts must have in place schemes for promoting racial equality. Such anti-discriminatory activity by the NHS and other public sector bodies exists in the context of the Human Rights Act (1998), which describes absolute, limited and qualified rights, and also reflects EU legislation (Tilki, 2006). The NHS has taken this seriously and has commissioned and implemented a number of initiatives relating to patients and staff, which can be accessed through a search of the NHS website (the abbreviation BME is used to represent Black and Minority Ethnic patients and staff).

Activity 4.4

In order to understand how insensitive cultural awareness can hamper good quality care, work through the case study exercises on the Transcultural Nursing website (www.culturediversity.org), which has a wealth of information about these issues.

There is no outline at the end of the chapter as the exercises on the website are self-explanatory.

C H A P T E R   S U M M A R Y

- We discussed the impact that the important early figures, Florence Nightingale and Mary Seacole, had on healthcare in their society. We noted that, while they overcame difficult personal circumstances, these were concerned with race and class, not gender, because in their society as well as ours caring is gendered and nursing is a gendered occupation.
- Gender inequalities have traditionally had an impact on the power relationships between nursing and medicine.
- The gender composition of medicine has changed recently, and this has altered this picture, but power inequality remains in the form of disparities in pay and status.
- The idea of culturally competent care was introduced towards the end of the chapter and we illustrated how important this is in delivering appropriate standards of care in a multicultural context.
- These are important ideas for nurses to understand as they affect how nursing roles have evolved, how nurses are treated in society and indicate how nurses must respond to cultural issues for individual patients and clients.

Activities: brief outline answers

4.1 Florence Nightingale and Mary Seacole (page 64)

- *What was the Victorian attitude towards women and how did they view their status and responsibilities?* Women in Victorian society were not equal in status to men, and were supposed to defer to men in all things apart from family and caring responsibilities. Victorian society could be extremely harsh to those who transgressed its norms.
- *What was the popular image of nurses and nursing at the time?* Nursing was a lower-class occupation and nurses were generally held to be drunken, rough and disreputable.

4.2 Gender inequalities (page 68)

- *Find out what the terms vocation and profession mean. Is nursing a vocation or a profession?* Generally, a vocation is held to be a 'calling', something that a person would undertake through a deep sense of personal conviction, religious belief or love of humanity. A profession has many definitions, largely concerned with having an expert body of knowledge, standing and status in the community, and with being responsible for decision making for people based on one's knowledge and skills. Nursing has traditionally been seen as a vocation and medicine more of a profession, although this is changing.
- *Compare the roles of Nurse Consultants to those of Hospital medical or surgical Consultants. What is it about their roles and responsibilities that*

means doctors earn more than nurses? One argument is that medicine requires greater skills and knowledge than nursing, and so doctors deserve to be paid more than nurses. A counter-argument is that doctors have an enshrined position within the NHS dating from when men were key decision makers and powerful people within society, and their greater pay illustrates a long-standing gender inequality between men and women.

Knowledge review

Having completed the chapter, how would you rate your knowledge of the following topics?

	Good	Adequate	Poor
1. Understanding of the caring culture and tradition in nursing including Florence Nightingale and Mary Seacole.			
2. An appreciation of how issues of gender can influence caring.			
3. An understanding of the distinction between 'caring for' and 'caring about'.			
4. An overview of caring in a diverse and multicultural context.			

Further reading

Davies, C (1995) *Gender and the Professional Predicament in Nursing.* Buckingham: Open University Press.

Essential reading.

Dossey, BM, Selanders, L, Beck D-M and Attewell, A (2005) *Florence Nightingale Today: Healing, leadership, global action.* Silver Spring, MD: American Nurses Association.

Kai, S (ed.) (2003) *Ethnicity, Health and Primary Care.* Oxford: Oxford University Press.

Nightingale, F (1969) *Notes on Nursing: What it is and what it is not.* New York: Dover Publications.

Papadopoulos, I (ed.) (2006) *Transcultural Health and Social Care: Development of culturally competent practitioners.* Oxford: Elsevier.

Seacole, M (1857) *Wonderful Adventures of Mrs Seacole in Many Lands.* London: James Blackwood.

Available online at http://digital.library.upenn.edu/women/seacole/adventures/adventures.html#VIII (accessed 28 March 2007).

Useful websites

http://tcn.sagepub.com *Journal of Transcultural Nursing* website.
www.culturediversity.org Transcultural Nursing website.
www.dh.gov.uk Department of Health website.
www.florence-nightingale-avenging-angel.co.uk Website of Hugh Small, a biographer of Nightingale.
www.florence-nightingale.co.uk/index.php Florence Nightingale Museum website.
www.florence-nightingale-foundation.org.uk Florence Nightingale Foundation website.
www.maryseacole.com Mary Seacole Centre for Nursing Practice website.
www.tcns.org Transcultural Nursing Society.
www2.uchsc.edu Jean Watson's website, originator of the Theory of Human Caring. Search the site for Jean Watson. Various interesting links.

Chapter 5

Evidence-based practice

Chapter aims

After reading this chapter you will be able to :

- understand the importance of research and evidence in nursing practice;
- begin to understand key quantitative and qualitative research approaches at a basic level;
- develop coherent clinical questions to use for literature searching;
- search electronic databases for research studies;
- begin to read studies in a critical manner.

Introduction

In this chapter, we are going to consider evidence-based practice (EBP). This development in healthcare decision making can enhance clinical effectiveness by allowing us to make judgements about which treatments and procedures work, rather than relying on custom and practice alone. In the second part of the chapter we will examine how to establish the credibility of evidence, both qualitative and quantitative.

Evidence-based practice

The importance of evidence-based practice

Evidence-based practice (EBP) is fundamental to recent government health reforms (Carnwell, 2000). It informs the provisions in NSFs, which set out what patients can expect from the NHS and the required standards and guidelines that nurses and other health professionals should work to in delivering care (DH, 1998b). Appraisal and synthesis of evidence is also a central element in the authoritative clinical guidelines produced by NICE. Quality improvement strategies also depend in part on using best evidence to achieve improvements in care and services (NHSE, 1999b). Rather than 'doing things as they have always been done around here', using EBP is crucial as it offers nurses and other HCPs the opportunity to investigate their practice and inform its development (Carnwell, 2000). From its birth in medicine, EBP has spread to many other professional and technical fields in a global movement; the underlying aim is to improve the effectiveness of decision making by making sure that decisions made by practitioners, managers and policy makers are based on sound rationale and use 'scientific approaches'. This is important for you as you undertake your programme of study as it helps you to understand research findings, and is likely to be increasingly so as your career progresses, your expertise develops and you become a decision maker in your chosen field: it is this expertise that your patients will expect and require.

There are many factors driving the need for EBP (Hek and Moule, 2006), such as:

- an explosion of evidence in many forms from sources such as academic and professional journals, on the internet and in other media;
- an emphasis on 'value for money' and the need to secure best value in treatment and care;
- adverse events and litigation in healthcare practice;
- increased access to information among patients and clients.

EBP should be a cyclical process (see Figure 5.1), in which research is assessed for its rigour, then linked with practitioners' expertise, causing EBP to be developed.

Figure 5.1: EBP as a cyclical process.

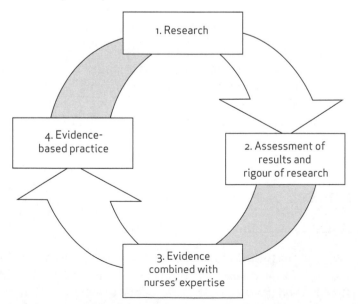

Source: Adapted from Critical Appraisal Skills Programme and the Health Care Libraries Unit (1999).

Definitions of evidence-based practice

EBP is: *the conscientious, explicit and judicious use of current best evidence in making decisions about the care of individual patients, and involves integrating individual clinical expertise with the best available clinical evidence from research findings* (Sackett et al., 1996). *EBP occurs when decisions that affect the care of patients are taken with regard to all valid, relevant information* (Hicks, 1997).

So, while there has always been research taking place into many aspects of treatment and care, the 'EBP project' recognises that research may be good in itself, but if it changes nothing it is not of much value in the real world of patient care. EBP therefore means undertaking the practical aspects of appraising and applying research for the benefit of patients, clients, staff and service delivery. There are five key steps by which individual nurses can identify their own clinical issues, find evidence and implement it in the clinical setting, thus making sure that they are practising EBP (Hek and Moule, 2006):

- Identify a problem from practice and turn it into a focused question.
- Search the literature to find the best available evidence.
- Appraise the evidence against set criteria to assess its rigour and usefulness.
- Apply the best evidence in line with the needs of patients and clients.
- Evaluate the use of evidence according to the impact of patients, clients and staff.

What constitutes evidence?

Explicit in EBP is the idea that some evidence is better than others. The following list illustrates this by showing the accepted '**hierarchy of evidence**': sources of evidence at the top of the list are accepted as 'better', meaning that they are more powerful, more authoritative, more credible and therefore likely to be more important in informing decision making than those further down the hierarchy (Hek and Moule, 2006):

1. Evidence from systematic reviews and meta-analyses including Cochrane systematic reviews and met-analyses.
2. Evidence from one or more randomised controlled trials.
3. Evidence from other quantitative studies.
4. Evidence from descriptive studies and qualitative research.
5. Evidence from expert committees or formal consensus methods.
6. Expert opinion.

The 'EBP project' has been widely accepted among HCPs, but there has been dissent in the literature (Hek and Moule, 2006). This focuses on several points:

- clinical guidelines can reduce clinical freedom and can be dangerous if followed without careful attention to the needs of individual patients;
- ethical dilemmas may be created for nurses if clinical guidelines conflict with their identification of patients' and clients' best interests;
- having a hierarchy of evidence (see the list above) means that EBP is implicitly

biased against qualitative research; this means that patient experiences are relegated to a lesser position in research terms, and may not even be researched;
- EBP is in fact decision making by statisticians, producing good statistics but not necessarily good practice.

Clinical effectiveness

This is concerned with using treatments or care that have been shown to work (are clinically effective, CE). It is important that what nurses do is effective, not least because the NHS is a publicly funded service and it would be financially wasteful, pointless and immoral for nurses to be using particular clinical interventions if they were known to be ineffective. Government and society need to be sure that practitioners' care maintains and improves health within the cash-limited resources of the NHS (NHSE, 1996, 1998a, b). There is an explicit link between EBP and CE, which is that nurses will use their clinical judgement to apply evidence in the best interests of patients and clients.

CE has been described as using the six Rs (Table 5.1): 'The right person, doing the right thing, the right way, in the right place, at the right time, with the right result.'

The six Rs link clinical effectiveness to providing quality care. They also show how CE differs from EBP because the need to use best evidence is placed in the context of the organisation and of patient satisfaction.

Table 5.1: Six Rs of clinical effectiveness.

The right **person**	Was the **person delivering the care** competent, with the right skills and knowledge?
The right **thing**	Was there **evidence to support the intervention**, and was the patient agreeable?
The right **way**	Was an intervention **used correctly**, with correct skills and competence, or to meet national guidelines and priorities?
The right **place**	Could the patient have been treated at home, or was there a **more appropriate place** based on specialist equipment or staff?
The right **time**	Was the intervention **timely** – would it have been more effective without a six-month wait?
The right **result**	Did it do **what was intended**?

Source: Adapted from Bury and Mead (1998).

Establishing credibility of evidence

A key aspect of EBP for nurses is about establishing the credibility of research reports, and to do this it is necessary to understand some basic research terminology. The following section is intended to introduce these concepts but does not fully describe them, and students should consult texts in the 'Further reading' section at the end of the chapter for more detailed explanations.

A distinction is drawn between quantitative and qualitative research because they start from very different premises about the world, are conducted using different concepts and methods, and are very different to read and to interpret.

Quantitative research

In general, researchers would choose a quantitative approach if they were seeking to answer well-defined questions such as 'What type of dressing heals leg ulcers the quickest?' or 'How many patients have leg ulcers in the community?' This is known as a *deductive approach*, where theories or questions are tested in real-life situations, and for Carter (2000) there is an emphasis on:

- objectivity (the researcher stands outside the situation);
- measurement (of different properties in participants called variables; these variables are analysed and presented using statistics);
- reductionism (complex phenomena can be reduced to numerical values and these values tested and compared statistically to answer important research questions).

Qualitative research

A qualitative approach would be preferred for a less structured, more exploratory type of question, such as 'What are patients' experiences of living with leg ulcers?' This is known as an *inductive approach*, where theories emerge from real-life situations, and there is an emphasis (Porter, 2000) on:

- subjectivity (researchers are generally more involved with participants, and may even have strong, pre-existing views on issues under study); researchers must make their ideas and values clear in their research reports, and this is called *reflexivity*;
- understanding and explanation (of participants' views by researchers, remaining truthful to their accounts; usually without numerical values and relying on text and themes from interviews);
- depth and prolonged engagement (people may be asked to give their views of issues in great depth over long periods of time, so complex ideas do not lose their meaning and context).

In all research studies, the type of question being asked is the first step and dictates the type of research approach taken.

Although there are many different research approaches in this section we will look at some of the most common. These are experimental designs and surveys (examples of quantitative research) and qualitative research concepts (including generic qualitative research based on interviews). Towards the end of the chapter there are exercises encouraging you to find examples of each, and undertake a brief critique of a paper from each category. 'Further reading' is indicated at the end of the chapter to add more depth to your understanding. Below is an activity to introduce you to some basic research terminology.

Activity 5.1

In order to begin to understand some important research terms in relation to quantitative and qualitative research, using the internet, textbooks from the 'Further reading' section and journal articles, look up and write a brief definition of the following terms.

General concepts

- Data
- Hawthorne effects
- Sampling

Quantitative concepts

- Generalisability
- Levels of measurement:
  o Nominal
  o Ordinal
  o Interval
- Mean
- Median
- Mode
- Reliability
- Statistics:
  o Descriptive statistics
  o Inferential statistics
- Statistical significance
- Validity
- Variables
- Independent variables
- Dependent variables

Activity 5.1 continued

Qualitative concepts

- Focus groups
- Themes
- Transcription
- Transferability
- Trustworthiness

Sample definitions (in alphabetical order) are to be found at the end of this chapter.

Quantitative research

Experimental designs: randomised controlled trials

An experimental approach involves setting up a research study in which the outcome is not known (Donnan, 2000). There will be comparisons between some characteristics of a group of participants experiencing some new treatment or procedure and those in another group who do not experience this new factor. In healthcare this is used to test a new treatment, medicine or procedure so that the researchers can establish whether it 'works' or not. They may have very strong suspicions based on their previous knowledge and/or the literature. They are setting out to demonstrate whether these are correct and are thus investigating their research question, also known as 'testing their hypothesis'.

For example, in developing a new drug treatment, pharmaceutical company researchers go through years of laboratory and animal-based testing before they are allowed to try it out on humans. In setting up a randomised controlled trial (RCT), researchers might have a good idea that the new medicine will work (they will have a research question or hypothesis that reflects that belief), and have satisfied an ethics committee that it will work. RCTs dominate thinking on what constitutes 'evidence' in healthcare research and are:

> *the gold standard for demonstrating in a rigorously scientific manner that a treatment or intervention is effective [and] the essential tool for a quantitative assessment of the efficacy of an intervention.*

(Donnan 2000, p175)

In essence, RCTs are a simple idea. Imagine there is a new treatment for high blood pressure (hypertension): the outcomes in the treatment group (those taking the drug) will be compared to those in the placebo group (those not taking the drug but an inert tablet that will have no clinical outcome). Researchers will measure by how much the treatment group's blood pressures decrease compared to the placebo group's blood pressures. (In the real world it would not be ethical to leave a group of hypertensive patients without treatment because of the potential health problems they would experience, so for safety and ethical reasons RCTs often evaluate a new treatment against 'normal care' as the control group. In this example, normal care would be existing antihypertensive medications, to try to demonstrate that the new treatment is a better option compared to existing methods.) Outcomes will be demonstrated using statistical techniques, searching for statistical significance in terms of the outcomes between the two groups. It may be the case that patients taking the new antihypertensive medication show a mean (or average) reduction in blood pressure, and that this is shown to be a statistically significant reduction compared to the control group. If this is the case, the researchers can claim that their new treatment 'works' and, provided the study has been set up and run in the appropriate scientific manner, their findings are generalisable to a larger population of hypertensive patients. The new drug would be shown to be clinically effective, and could be used more widely. (This does not always occur as NICE may not recommend the medication for use on the grounds of cost-effectiveness.)

However, it is the extent of control that is essential. Both groups must be very similar in characteristics, so that, if there is a treatment effect before and after the new intervention, it must be *only* the intervention that caused it (not age, sex, class, race, income, or any other variables). In this way, the researchers can be confident that it is the active compound in the new antihypertensive and nothing else that causes the beneficial outcomes.

Essential features of a randomised controlled trial

For a study to be a true experiment, the following features apply (Donnan, 2000).

- Comparison and control groups are required to test a hypothesis: variables will be manipulated and outcomes assessed. In an RCT, the group to which participants are allocated is the independent variable, and the outcome is the dependent variable: in our antihypertensive trial, treatment or control groups are the independent variables, and the impact on blood pressure is the dependent variable.
- Sampling and sample size: a sample is a small number of eligible participants from a larger population. These people will participate in the trial, because it would be impossible to treat all the UK hypertensives with the new drug. The size of the sample is important and is decided at the planning stage and acknowledged in research reports. Many statistical tests are more reliable and powerful in their ability to detect differences between groups with larger numbers (thousands rather than tens); authors should include a paragraph stating that they recruited enough participants into the study for differences to be accurately measured (a sample size estimate or power calculation).
- Eligibility of subjects: there should be clear protocols with inclusion and exclusion criteria such as age and sex for all participants, to ensure that those enrolled in the study are appropriate.
- Fully informed consent, without which the study would be unethical: researchers are required to submit their potential studies to an ethics committee, and without its approval the study cannot go ahead (information on arrangements in the NHS can be found online at www.nres.npsa.nhs.uk).

- Randomisation: from the recruited sample eligible subjects will be randomised into two groups. This means that participants are randomly allocated to either the treatment or the control group to avoid potential biases if they were chosen for each group by researchers. The research and control groups should be similar enough in composition after randomisation to enable meaningful comparison.
- Blinding of treatment: it should be impossible for patients, staff and researchers to know who is receiving the new treatment and who is not. This is to avoid bias in the findings if participants were treated differently because of the group they were in, even if this happens unconsciously.
- Analysis of differences between research or control groups: using appropriate statistical tests and software (a common package is SPSS, the Statistical Package for the Social Sciences).

A study that does not meet all these criteria in some way may be discussed as a quasi-experimental design, which generally means that the researchers have made compromises in the study design in order to investigate their hypotheses. These studies are therefore weaker than more rigorous RCTs. Common reasons for this are that it is impossible to produce a convincing placebo, or it is not possible to ensure adequate blinding for a study, or it is not possible for the groups to be set up with complete equivalence. (Ethical approval will still need to be applied for and obtained, and the researchers would need to discuss limitations of their study in published articles.)

Limitations of RCTs

No research study is perfect! All have strengths and weaknesses, and studies will show these in some measure. Donnan (2000) has outlined some of these for RCTs.

- Non-compliance: do participants actually take the new tablets?
- Dropout rates: this means that participants are lost to the study, so clinical outcomes cannot be assessed. This may be because of side effects of the new treatment, which are also not documented if participants drop out. Patients may leave the study voluntarily, or may pass away or move away from the area.
- Quantitative measures only give figures: these may be statistically and/or clinically significant; and they can be extremely difficult for the non-specialist to interpret, making many papers dense and impenetrable to read. Consequently, readers must rely on the authors' or their statisticians' interpretation of results. It is not a flaw if a study reports no statistically significant differences between active and control groups in an RCT. It is as clinically useful to know that a new treatment or procedure does not work as it is to know that it does: if it does not work, there is no need to introduce it!
- Potential Hawthorne effects: it is entirely possible that groups gain some benefit just because something new is being done to them, as the mind can produce all kinds of physical and psychological responses to treatments and placebos. The Hawthorne effect is thus defined as occurring when an effect noted in a research study could occur because participants know they are

involved in the study (Hek and Moule, 2006). This is why a control group is needed, to assess whether the new treatment works over and above any Hawthorne effects there might be.

- RCTs tell us nothing about the patient's experience: new anti-hypertensives might lower the blood pressure but, if they make patients feel so ill that they would not take them, this would not be discovered in an RCT.

Research examples

Below are three examples of RCTs in nursing from two leading UK nursing journals, *The Journal of Advanced Nursing* and *The Journal of Clinical Nursing* (Blackwell Publishing). Unfamiliar terminology and key concepts are highlighted in bold type, and you should read around these concepts more thoroughly using the 'Further reading' at the end of the chapter (a good place to start looking for introductory ideas is Jupp (2006), *The Sage Dictionary of Social Research Methods*).

Cooke et al. (2005) examined the effect of music on preoperative anxiety in day surgery. They sought to test the hypothesis that people who listened to music during their preoperative care experience less anxiety than patients receiving 'routine care' (meaning whatever happens normally on the unit in day surgery). This was their study aim.

They argued that the research was necessary, because previous research had indicated that music can be effective in reducing anxiety, but that previous studies had been limited and flawed in ways that called their findings into question. This was the background to their study.

In order to test their hypothesis, they conducted a randomized controlled trial to discover whether it was indeed the case that music reduced anxiety, and they did this by allocating patients to one of three groups (these are the independent variables): an intervention group (who received music), a placebo group (who wore headphones but did not listen to music), and a control group (who received routine care).

Participants were tested before and after listening to music using an existing measure of anxiety (the State-Trait Anxiety Inventory). This was their method of data collection, and they analyzed the data for statistically significant differences between the groups using various statistical tests.

Their study found that music did reduce the anxiety of participants in the intervention group. This result was a statistically significant difference between the intervention (music) group and the placebo and control groups. The authors concluded that music should be used as a nursing intervention for preoperative anxiety associated with day surgery.

de Wit, R and van Dam, F (2001) conducted a study investigating the effects of a pain education programme (PEP) for patients and their district nurses. This was the **study aim**, and they argued that it was necessary because there are no studies on whether such education can make a difference to patients' pain.

They enrolled 104 patients and 115 district nurses in a **prospective, longitudinal, randomized controlled study**. The concepts they sought to investigate were:

- district nurses' care provision;
- satisfaction with pain treatment;
- how far nurses and patients agreed in their estimation of patients' pain.

The authors used a variety of existing **valid and reliable measures** to assess these variables (by **collecting data**), and various techniques to demonstrate **statistical significance** (perform **statistical analysis**).

The study found the following results relating to the variables under study:

- district nurses' care provision: only 36 per cent of nurses were informed about patients' pain by hospital sources;
- satisfaction with pain treatment: pain was the subject under discussion in 76 per cent of visits, but nurses provided only a few pain relief interventions;
- how far nurses and patients agreed in their estimation of patients' pain: those nurses in the intervention group (receiving the PEP) better estimated patients' pain and were more satisfied about patients' pain treatment, but no differences were found in their assessment of patients' pain relief compared to the control group (who were not offered the PEP).

The authors concluded that the PEP can have some impact on district nurses' pain care, but that in their study location plays only a small role in pain treatment.

Plastow et al. (2001) conducted a study to examine the effectiveness of a method of removing lice from children's hair (called 'bug busting') with the usual method of applying lotion. They argued that there was inconclusive evidence to indicate which worked best, and therefore that their study was necessary.

They conducted a **pilot study randomized controlled trial** with small numbers of children, who were assigned to two **intervention groups**: one

Research examples continued

group was treated with phenothrin lotion (a special preparation to kill parasites), and the other group (the bug busting group) had their hair combed using special combs and ordinary hair conditioner. The key **dependent variable** was the number of live lice at day 14.

The authors found that those in the bug busting group had **statistically significant (p=0.05)** total eradication of lice compared to the lotion group and they concluded that bug busting is effective in managing head lice infestation.

Survey designs

A survey design is a very different quantitative approach to that described above. There will still be research questions, and hypotheses may still be tested, but there are no treatment or control groups. A survey, therefore, is not an experimental design. There are two main types of survey, one with the purpose of finding out information to describe a current situation (a *descriptive* survey), and the other to explain relationships between variables (an *explanatory* survey) (Hek and Moule, 2006). Questionnaires are usually used for these purposes, posted with a stamped addressed envelope or, increasingly, emailed with a return address.

There will be inclusion and exclusion criteria for the study, and a sampling frame will be constructed drawing a representative sample from a larger population. For example, if we wanted to find out attitudes of female nurses towards the practicalities of childcare arrangements when working for the NHS, we would make sure our sample was made up of female nurses with children who work in the NHS, so each property would be an inclusion criterion for our study. As there are several hundred thousand nurses on the NMC register in the UK, we could not possibly send them all a questionnaire, so we would take a sample and send only these nurses our questionnaire. Their returns would be our data, and we could analyse these data accordingly. If we wanted to describe the numbers who were satisfied or dissatisfied we could say that (perhaps) 67 per cent were satisfied with their experiences of childcare provision, based on their questionnaire responses.

If we wanted to go further in an explanatory survey we could use statistical tests to look for relationships in the data. Perhaps we might be interested in examining whether those earning the highest wages were more satisfied than those on low wages, particularly if the literature indicated that the high earners could afford more flexible childcare provision to fit in with their shift patterns. If our results indicated that this was the case, there would be a relationship between income and satisfaction with childcare provision, known as a *correlation*. This would be demonstrated by showing statistically significant findings. In this example, the income would be the independent variable, and the attitude towards childcare would be the dependent variable; increasing income would be seen to predict potentially greater satisfaction with childcare provision (see Figure 5.2 which indicates that as income increases, so does satisfaction with childcare).

Figure 5.2:   Correlation between income and satisfaction with childcare.

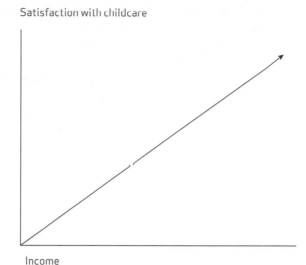

Strengths of surveys

- Large numbers of people can be reached cheaply and easily. Samples from a population can be used, and sample size estimation should be acknowledged. The results are generalisable if the sampling is undertaken correctly.
- Questionnaires are easy to draw up. However, in more sophisticated research the validity and reliability of the questionnaire must be assessed, so that, if researchers simply invent their own questionnaire, they don't run the risk of it being poor, biased and not measuring meaningful properties in the sample. Many survey tools, or ratings scales, are now available that have undergone processes of rigorous testing and development. Good surveys, therefore, are accurate and objective, and have been tested to demonstrate validity and reliability.
- There are usually few ethical considerations involved in distributing surveys. People can choose to complete them or not in the privacy of their own homes or workplaces, meaning also that confidentiality and anonymity can be high.

Limitations of surveys

Although easy, surveys are not problem-free. The following problems have been identified by Atkinson (2000).

- Non-response rates: researchers undertaking postal survey designs have to work hard with reminders and second mailings to get over 50 per cent response rates. If only half the people reply, the researcher has no way of knowing what the others think. Those who respond may feel very strongly about the issues and therefore the findings would be biased because neutral beliefs are not represented.

- Reductionism: questionnaires reduce complex concepts to numerical values, often in Likert-type scales where a respondent may be asked to rate their attitudes to something complex and personal on a scale from 1–5, where 1 = very dissatisfied and 5 = very satisfied. These scales can be used to measure intimate, personal attributes or reactions to events, and they therefore reduce these complex phenomena to numerical values. This makes it possible to do simple comparisons and/or run complex statistical procedures, but this is unlikely to capture the essence of an event as each individual experienced it.
- Sampling errors are common, which limits the results' generalisability.
- As they are often self-report (that is, people fill them out themselves), responses can vary due to date and time of completion, or to strength of feeling because of factors outside the control of the study. Also, the researchers do not know who is actually responding.
- Respondents may give the answers they think are required.
- Respondents may give the answers they think will portray them in the most favourable light.

Research examples

Below are three recent examples of surveys in nursing from *The Journal of Advanced Nursing*. Make sure to read around the highlighted concepts using the suggested 'Further reading' at the end of the chapter.

Griffin and Melby (2006) conducted a study examining nurses', doctors' and GPs' attitudes about developing advanced Nurse Practitioner services within a hospital emergency department. **This was the aim of the study**. They argued that such advanced nursing roles have emerged in emergency care in many different countries, but that, having begun with nurses offering a service for 'minor' problems and progressed to all areas of clinical care, there is no consensus about post-holders' roles, lines of accountability and educational needs.

In order to **collect data**, a survey was carried out using a **questionnaire survey**. A **Likert rating scale** was developed to measure attitudes and collect **demographic variables**, with two **open-ended questions** allowing **respondents** to elaborate. All GPs, emergency nurses and doctors in one health board in the Republic of Ireland were sent the questionnaire. This was the researchers' **sampling frame**: 25 emergency nurses, 13 emergency doctors and 69 GPs were asked to take part.

Questionnaires were returned from 74·8 per cent. This was the **response rate**. Respondents were positive towards the development of an advanced Nurse Practitioner service, although GPs were less so.

The authors concluded that a multidisciplinary approach and accredited educational programmes are required.

Research examples continued

Douglas et al. (2006) report a study, which investigated health visitors' and practice nurses' attitudes and practice concerning advising patients about physical activity. This was the **study aim**.

The authors argue that obesity is increasing at the same time as physical activity levels are decreasing. Primary healthcare professionals can promote physical activity within their local populations, but few studies exist which examine nurses' experiences of such work.

In order to **collect data** a **questionnaire survey** was sent to 630 **potential respondents**. The **response rate** was 63 per cent.

Their study found that over 80 per cent of health visitors and practice nurses were very likely or likely to recommend all patients to exercise, but only about 10 per cent described correctly the current recommendations of 30 minutes of physical activity five times weekly. These were their **results**. They concluded that nurses and health visitors were enthusiastic about promoting physical activity for clients.

Gray et al. (2005) surveyed patient satisfaction with, and experiences of, being treated with antipsychotic medication. These were the **study aims**.

They argue that patient satisfaction is an important issue in contemporary healthcare practice, but that there is limited literature on the issue of antipsychotic treatment.

To **collect data**, **a cross-sectional survey** was carried out with patients who were not in hospital but were under active treatment. This was their **sampling frame**, and included 75 schizophrenic patients. Their **response rate** was 39 per cent. Patients reported satisfaction with their medication and communication with mental health professionals, but did not feel involved in treatment decisions, took medication because they were told to, and were not warned about side-effects. They concluded that although patient satisfaction was high, side-effects were not being managed effectively by professionals. Further research was recommended.

Validity and reliability in quantitative research

In quantitative research, rigour, validity and reliability are important concepts in establishing whether the study is a good one and therefore that the results are important sources of evidence for practice. They come from a 'scientific' approach to data collection and analysis: the researcher is objective and detached, responding only to the 'facts' or patterns produced by the underlying 'laws' of nature.

- **Rigour**: the extent to which a study has been carried out using an appropriate and 'scientific' method.
- **Reliability**: the degree of consistency with which an instrument measures the property it is supposed to be measuring. A weighing scale that measured a bag of sugar at 2kg on one attempt and 3kg on the next (and so on) would not be a reliable instrument. So, reliability is associated with the stability, consistency or dependability of the measuring tool. It is also associated with its accuracy.
- **Validity**: the degree to which an instrument measures what it is supposed to be measuring. How do we know that a questionnaire developed to measure occupational stress is not actually measuring something else (like job satisfaction)? There are a number of statistical tests that can be performed to measure these properties in a questionnaire or other measuring instrument (Carter and Porter, 2000).

Qualitative research

Qualitative research is entirely different from quantitative research. Researchers may have questions that they are interested in finding out about, but there are not clearly formulated hypotheses as there are in quantitative research. This means that theories are developed out of the situation by the research study, rather than being tested experimentally, and this is called an *inductive approach* (Hek and Moule, 2006). Generally, the intention is to find out about an issue, using the participants' own voices and opinions to gain in-depth understanding.

Qualitative research studies usually take place in local settings, with small numbers (tens rather than hundreds), and researchers are frequently much closer to the participants than they are in quantitative research. Objectivity is not such an issue, neither is generalisability, and different criteria other than validity and reliability may be used to evaluate qualitative research (Carter and Porter, 2000).

As it is inductive, qualitative research is useful where little is known about an issue, where little research has already been conducted, or where researchers are seeking to build a picture of what issues might be relevant in preparation for developing ideas or measurement tools for larger-scale quantitative research. In mixed methods research, a study might use both qualitative and quantitative methods to gain an understanding of issues from different perspectives, and data would be analysed together using techniques of triangulation (Williamson, 2004).

Qualitative research has a long history and tradition, being based in various schools of philosophy and political ideology. Major approaches and associated terms are listed below (Hek and Moule, 2006).

- **Action research**: specifically designed to change practice in an area, so is well suited to nursing research. A 'spiral' framework of planning, action, evaluation and further planning is used, and there is an emphasis on close collaboration between researcher and subjects (rather than the researcher in a powerful and dominant position; Williamson et al., 2004).
- **Ethnography**: an approach that involves the researcher being in some way part of participants' setting or context. In classic twentieth-century forms,

ethnographers were anthropologists studying peoples in very different societies from their own European ones, and so prolonged exposure was required. However, in healthcare research it is not necessary to live with patients for a year to conduct an ethnographic study.

- **Grounded theory**: an interview- and/or observation-based technique that allows the development of knowledge about a subject where there is little existing currently. The researcher returns to the field to test and refine ideas generated from initial interviews and continues until no new data are generated (known as saturation). This is a commonly used approach that requires close attention to technique, and has a potentially open-ended time scale.
- **Phenomenology**: a research technique that studies the participants' lived experiences of events and circumstances. Although deeply rooted in philosophical traditions, phenomenology is used in nursing to study clinical issues and are important in forming our understanding of patient care and how to improve it.

Generic qualitative research

When conducting qualitative research studies using the methodologies referred to above, it is necessary to adhere closely to their underlying philosophical and procedural principles, and these may be logistically difficult or time-consuming. As a result it is becoming more common to see qualitative research studies where authors do not claim allegiance to any particular school of thought, meaning that qualitative techniques of data collection are used to conduct what is called 'generic qualitative research' (Caelli et al., 2003). There are many acceptable methods of data collection: key ones are listed below (these methods of data collection may also be used in the research approaches mentioned above).

- **In-depth interviews**: these can be with individuals or in groups, and are generally unstructured or semi-structured. Individual interviews are usually conducted face-to-face between the researcher and a participant, either in the clinical setting or at home. Focus groups offer the opportunity to talk to participants in a less threatening environment, and to access a range of views based on the interactions within the groups. Interviews are usually semi-structured but occasionally researchers administer a more structured schedule of questioning. Telephone interviews can be used to access busy clinical staff who would not otherwise attend interviews. Potential problems are non-attendance, 'leading' of participants by researchers' questions, and dominant characters overwhelming the discussion in focus groups.
- **Participant observation**: this is a classic qualitative technique that allows the researcher to enter into the participants' world. It is not usually taped or videoed and relies on the researcher's interpretation of events. Problems include that it is time-consuming; that the researchers' presence can influence participants' behaviour; that the findings are the interpretations of a single researcher (although two observers might prevent this overt bias); and that, when done covertly, it is ethically dubious.

Research examples

Below are three recent examples of qualitative research in nursing from two leading UK nursing journals, *The Journal of Advanced Nursing* and *The Journal of Clinical Nursing*. The first study is a phenomenological enquiry, the second uses grounded theory and the third takes a generic qualitative approach where data are collected in focus groups. Read around the highlighted concepts using the suggested 'Further reading' at the end of the chapter.

Broussard's (2005) study aimed to understand women's experiences of bulimia nervosa, arguing that, although much scientific evidence focuses on physical aspects of the illness, there is little published research on women's personal experiences, and so the study would help professionals to provide sensitive care.

Phenomenology was used to guide **data collection and analysis**. Thirteen bulimics were interviewed and kept personal diaries.

Broussard found four themes :

- isolating self, as a result of bulimic women's secret practices;
- living in fear, as a result of negative reactions of others;
- being at war with the mind, as a result of fear of gaining weight; and
- pacifying the brain, as a result of feeling guilty for eating and subsequent vomiting.

The author concludes that appreciation of bulimic women's perspectives could enable better understanding of bulimia, its aetiology, and treatment alternatives.

McCaughan and McKenna (2007) studied how patients newly diagnosed with cancer sought information in the immediate post diagnosis period.

They used a **grounded theory** approach to data collection and analysis and interviewed a **theoretical sample** of 27 newly diagnosed patients in their own homes. They developed a **substantive theory**, which describes newly diagnosed cancer patients' experience as moving through:

- 'being traumatized' by the diagnosis;
- to a phase of trying to 'take it on';
- through to 'taking control'.

McCaughan and McKenna provide a **theoretical framework** to understand patients' changing needs and their efforts to regain control over their lives, which they describe as a journey of *never-ending making sense*.

The authors conclude that the study **findings** provide nurses with a framework for their information-giving and to assist patients with their efforts to regain control over their lives.

Hutchings et al. (2005) explored how decisions are made concerning the number of student nurses that can be supported in clinical practice. This was the **study aim**, and the **objective** was to identify factors that are taken into consideration in the decision-making process.

This research was set in the context of increasing numbers of students as a result of expansion of the UK NHS, which had implications for the quality of placement learning in clinical placements.

Data were collected in three **focus group interviews**. Participants were recruited by **purposive sampling**, and analysis identified three themes from across the three groups. The themes were:

- capacity issues;
- enhancing support in practice; and
- issues impacting on learning in practice.

Hutchings et al. concluded that student-support decisions are complex, with a multitude of dimensions, and that educational staff are needed to support learning in practice.

Rigour and interpretation in qualitative research

In qualitative research, concepts of validity and reliability are more difficult to clarify, because of the researcher's closeness to the subjects and the attempt to elicit new knowledge rather than test theories. Thus qualitative research is frequently referred to as providing *interesting stories* (Monti and Tingen, 1999), relating only to one situation or circumstance, and cannot be applied to other settings. It is also criticised for a lack of rigour, validity and reliability. However, some argue that these concepts are not relevant in qualitative research, because the methods of data collection and underlying philosophy are so different (Cutcliffe and McKenna, 1999; Carter and Porter, 2000).

Trustworthiness and qualitative research

'Trustworthiness' is frequently debated in the literature on qualitative research, and is proposed as a qualitative researchers' alternative to the quantitative concepts of validity and reliability. Trustworthiness has four elements (Lincoln and Guba, 1984).

- **Credibility**: research should be undertaken so that readers can believe in it, so that it is clear that the findings have not been made up, and so that any biases have been acknowledged. To achieve this, certain criteria are necessary.
  - o 'Prolonged engagement' (long-term interaction between researcher and participants). This should give depth of understanding. Triangulation (using

more than one source of evidence, paradigm or data collection method to get a fuller picture of the issue under study) will also enhance credibility.

- o Peer debriefing, which involves researchers discussing and defending interpretations with colleagues who are not so close to the research and who can give a disinterested perspective.
- o Searching for disconfirming evidence (can the findings and their interpretation be questioned by any aspects of the data?).
- o Member checks (findings and their interpretation should be scrutinised by those who participated in the study).
- o Referential adequacy, which means allowing others to compare findings with portions of the data set aside for that purpose.
- **Transferability**: what is the relevance of the findings to other settings? Qualitative researchers do not produce generalisable findings because their work does not aim to prove a theory that can be applied to everyone in a population; they do not use appropriate sampling techniques or statistical methods. Qualitative work is context-bound: it is a product of the situation and circumstances in which it was conducted and is therefore unique to that setting. For qualitative work to be relevant to other readers, they must be able to decide if the context matches their own setting, so details of this must be given (*thick description* (Lincoln and Guba, 1984, p316)).
- **Dependability**: data should be stable over time and location, and internal audits should be available. Thus prolonged engagement is necessary to assess whether findings change over time.
- **Confirmability**: the same conclusions should be reached independently by researchers. Interview transcripts should produce the same themes if analysed by two or more people, and disagreements about their interpretation should be resolvable. There should be an audit trail available to do this, and potential issues of bias should be outlined so that they can be taken into account.

Searching for evidence and critical appraisal

Activity 5.2

So that you can have some practice at searching electronic databases and working out clinical questions that are relevant to your practice, in this section you are going to search for evidence on a clinical issue that interests you.

Sackett et al. (1997) use the formula PICO to establish a focused clinical question. PICO stands for:

Population
Intervention
Comparison
Outcome.

- So, start by defining the population: in whom are you interested? Is it student nurses; people with leg ulcers; people with diabetes? You may want to add in other characteristics such as age, sex, other diseases and so on to limit your question.

WRITE DOWN YOUR POPULATION

- Next, write down an intervention (or exposure) of interest. Are you interested in diabetic men who smoke cigarettes (an exposure), or different types of leg ulcer dressings, or different treatment regimes (interventions)?

WRITE DOWN YOUR INTERVENTION

- The next step is to work out a comparison (this will only apply in experimental studies). So, are you interested in particular types of diabetic therapies, or in different bandaging techniques for leg ulcer dressings?

WRITE DOWN YOUR COMPARISON

- Finally, outcomes: think about what you want to know from the above three steps. It is likely that papers you find will be quite specific in their outcomes, but you may not be able to define these so clearly at the outset.

WRITE DOWN YOUR OUTCOMES

Having completed the PICO exercise you now have a clinical question requiring an answer from the literature; you now have a series of search terms that you can use for searching electronic databases.

Detailed instruction on literature searching is outside the scope of this book but is usually offered to CFP students in induction events and early theoretical modules. If this is not the case, please approach the subject librarian at your university for further help.

Start by putting in your broad population heading. If numerous search 'hits' are found, you can limit your search using the terms you have written down under 'intervention', 'comparison' and 'outcomes'.

It is likely that you will find a body of evidence on your topic. If not this is an indication that primary research has not been conducted in the area, or it may mean that you need to rethink your question or refine your search terms.

As you have worked on an issue that interests you, there are no right and wrong answers, and no outline at the end of the chapter.

Critical appraisal

Critical appraisal is something we do every day when we make choices between competing courses of action or purchases (Hek and Moule, 2006). It is an essential part of EBP in that it allows us to make judgements about the value of research studies. Some research studies may be very good, and some may not be so good; some are exemplary and some are fatally flawed.

So how do you tell which studies are worth using to guide clinical practice or not? The process by which this is carried out is known as *critical appraisal*. Bodies such as NICE critically appraise research literature and draw up recommendations known as clinical guidelines to indicate good standards of care. In addition, techniques such as systematic review (a rigorous process of finding everything that has been written on a topic) and meta-analysis (constructing an overview of the literature) are undertaken by bodies such as the Cochrane Collaboration. The Cochrane Collaboration describes itself as an independent international organisation, which makes available up-to-date, accurate information about the effects of healthcare treatments and interventions (see www.cochrane.org for further information, where you will also be able to search for topics of interest). The findings it produces are authoritative and, as we have seen (see page 100), constitute the top of the hierarchy of evidence. However, while these national and international developments are important, this does not preclude every nurse from taking an interest in the research literature in areas of care for which they are responsible: indeed, all nurses *should* be using the literature to inform their practice, and this is a skill that can be learned by all.

Critical appraisal does not necessarily mean 'criticism', but as no research studies are perfect it is likely that you will find some queries about the evidence you have found using the PICO exercise (see Activity 5.2). Various critical appraisal frameworks exist, and they give you tools by which you can assess your studies in detail. References for further reading in critical appraisal and frameworks are at the end of the chapter.

Activity 5.3

This activity is intended to begin to familiarise you with the structure and key aspects of research reports (rather than detailed critical appraisal), noting queries and issues in studies. In this exercise you are asked to:

- Select two research studies from an electronic database search after using the PICO exercise to define a question and related search terms: one study should be an RCT and one a qualitative study;
- Read each paper once, then read them through again; write down answers to the following questions.

Study aims and research questions

- What are the aims of study?
- What are the research questions?
- For the RCT, are there hypotheses to be tested?

Literature review

- Is a range of up-to-date sources cited?
- Does the literature cited seem to be supporting only the authors' points of view (giving a biased perspective)?
- Does the literature explain why the research is necessary?
- Does the literature indicate that there are gaps in current knowledge, which the study seeks to fill?

Methodology

- What is the study design?
- How have the researchers undertaken sampling? Can you identify any issues that might introduce bias into the sample?
- What are the methods of data collection? (What techniques have the researchers used to get information from the participants?)
- How have the researchers analysed the data? Using percentages, statistics or themes based on text?

Results/findings

- What are the key results or findings and how are they presented? Are they in numerical form or in the form of text?
- In the RCT, can you identify how the researchers have indicated statistical significance? Do the results support or reject the research questions/hypotheses?
- In the qualitative study, can you identify how the researchers have sought to convince you that their findings are not simply 'interesting stories'? Are the findings credible to you as a reader?

Discussion and conclusions

- Do the authors list any strengths and weaknesses of their study? In your opinion are there any others that they have not listed?
- Do they discuss their findings in relation to the literature?
- Do they highlight areas that require changes to practice, or to education, or to further research?

Implications for practice

- For the RCT, has a rigorous, scientific approach been taken? Is it generalisable to a wider population?
- For the qualitative study, is it trustworthy and credible? Is it transferable to other settings?

Activity 5.3 continued

Based on your reading of both the research studies and thinking about your current clinical areas, can you identify the relevance of the studies? Is the clinical area adhering to their results or findings; can you identify areas where care could be improved by implementing the findings from the studies or their recommendations?

Your answers will depend on the papers you find, so there is no outline answer at the end of the chapter.

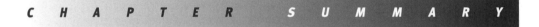

C H A P T E R   S U M M A R Y

- EBP is an increasingly important concept in all healthcare practice, and has the support of government through various policy drivers. Every nurse should be aware of the evidence base for their practice and should aim to be practising using the best available evidence. There is a clear hierarchy of evidence, with systematic reviews and meta analysis at the top of this hierarchy.
- Research findings can be complex and difficult to interpret, but at the CFP stage of a programme students should be familiar with how to outline key search terms, how to search for evidence using electronic databases, and with some of the key concepts used in quantitative and qualitative research such as randomised controlled trials, surveys and qualitative approaches. This chapter has briefly outlined some of these key concepts.
- It is important at CFP level that students are able to begin critically analysing evidence that they might find, and this chapter has suggested a basic format for structuring this critique.
- These are important ideas for nurses to understand as they provide a structure for learning about and improving clinical practice.

Activity: brief outline answer

5.1 Sample definitions of basic concepts (pages 84–5)

Data Collections of observations or text from people participating in the study (thus data is always a plural term, *these data*).

Focus groups These take place when about 5–8 people are brought together by a researcher to discuss an issue in depth. Group dynamics are paramount.

Generalisability The extent to which findings from a study can be said to apply to a larger population; underlying principle of some quantitative research.

Hawthorne effects The effect that can be observed in participants simply because they are enrolled in a research study. Hawthorne effects were originally discovered when researchers investigating factory workers' productivity found that different lighting in the work environment increased it; the point being that, whatever the researchers did to the lighting, even when they did nothing, productivity increased. They concluded that simply being involved in the study improved the workers' productivity.

Levels of measurement:
- nominal: indicates differences or similarities in data only, e.g. yes/no, male/female;
- ordinal: scale where size of intervals is not known or not equal; measures 'more' or 'less', e.g. good, fair, bad;
- interval: scale of equal interval, e.g. temperature (°C) or income.

Mean   The 'average' figure in a data set.

Median   The middle number in a data set. This would show how many numbers were above and how many below the middle number.

Mode   The number that comes up most frequently; if there are two numbers that come up, the data would be bimodal.

Reliability   The extent to which a data collection tool measures a property repeatedly over time.

Sampling   The process of taking a small number of participants from a population (all people with a certain property, which may be too large a number to take part in a study). The sample should represent that population in some way.

Statistical significance   The extent to which a result is 'true' in the sense that it represents a 'real' relationship between variables rather than an accidental or coincidental finding. This is demonstrated in research reports in two ways:
- p values (p meaning probability): a value may be written as $p=0.05$, meaning that there is a 5 per cent chance that the results in the sample are there by accident ($p=0.01$ is therefore only a 1 per cent chance of the results being a 'fluke'; even better than $p=0.05$);
- confidence intervals (CIs): these describe how reliable results are by indicating a range of values within which readers can be 95 per cent confident that the true result from the test undertaken in a sample lies for a population. The narrower the CI, the greater confidence there is about this result.

Statistics   The treatment of numerical data to find relationships between variables. Can be either:
- descriptive: methods used to describe data in simple terms (such as mean, median and mode); these could be presented in a series of graphs and tables;
- inferential: these draw inferences or predictions about relationships of interest in the data, such as differences between groups, or correlations.

Themes   These are constructed from the text of recorded interviews. Researchers will repeatedly read the interview transcripts and will construct themes using one of several recognised methods, depending on the type of qualitative research they are conducting.

Transcription   The process of typing a recorded interview so that the text can be analysed for themes.

Transferability   The qualitative term for generalisability, meaning how research findings can be applied to others in a similar setting. As there can be no statistical generalisation in qualitative research, transferability indicates if the research is useful or of interest to others; in part, the reader's judgement.

Trustworthiness Used by qualitative researchers instead of validity, indicating that the findings represent reality.

Validity The extent to which a data collection tool measures what it is intended to measure.

Variables Properties of participants that researchers are interested in finding out more about, particularly the relationships they have with other variables. These can be:

- independent: a property that each participant has independently of anything else in the study (age, gender); the cause rather than the effect; a property that is manipulated in experimental designs to assess its impact among participants;
- dependent: influenced by other variables, including the independent variable.

Knowledge review

Now you have completed this chapter, how would you rate your knowledge of the following topics?

	Good	Adequate	Poor
1. Understanding the importance of research and evidence in nursing practice.			
2. Beginning to understand key quantitative and qualitative research approaches.			
3. Formulating coherent clinical questions to use for literature searching.			
4. Searching electronic databases for research studies.			
5. Beginning to read studies in a critical manner.			

Further reading

Those that are all in bold contain critical appraisal frameworks.

Cormack, D (ed.) (2006) *The Research Process in Nursing*, 5th edition. Oxford: Blackwell Science.
Good introductory text.

Hek, G and Moule, P (2006) Making Sense of Research: An introduction for health and social care practitioners. London: Sage.
Good introductory text for this level.

Jupp, V (2006) *The Sage Dictionary of Social Research Methods.* London: Sage.
Brief definitions of much of the terminology employed by researchers when reporting research reports. A good place to start looking for the highlighted terms from the research example papers.

Parahoo, K (2006) *Nursing Research: Process and issues,* 2nd edition. Basingstoke: Palgrave Macmillan.
Very good general text.

Polit, DF and Back, CT (2006) *Essentials of Nursing Research Methods, Appraisal, and Utilization,* 2nd edition. London: Lippincott, Williams and Wilkins.

Wright, DB (2002) *First Steps in Statistics.* London: Sage.

Useful websites

http://ebn.bmj.com/ *Evidence Based Nursing* online journal.
www.cochrane.co.uk Cochrane Collaboration.
www.joannabriggs.edu.au/ Joanna Briggs Institute for Evidence Based Nursing.
www.jr2.ox.ac.uk/bandolier/ *Bandolier* (electronic monthly magazine on evidence-based healthcare).
www.man.ac.uk/rcn RCN Research and Development Coordinating Centre.
www.nice.org.uk National Institute for Health and Clinical Excellence (NICE).
www.phru.nhs.uk/casp/casp.htm CASP: aims to enable individuals to develop the skills to find and make sense of research evidence, helping them to put knowledge into practice. CASP's workshops and resources are in three main areas: finding research evidence, appraising research evidence, and acting on research evidence. CASP critical appraisal tools can be found at www.phru.nhs.uk/casp/critical_appraisal_tools.htm.
www.psychiatry.ox.ac.uk/cebmh/ Centre for Evidence Based Mental Health.
www.shef.ac.uk/~scharr School of Health and Related Research (SCHARR).
www.tripdatabase.com/index.html Trip Plus: brings together all the 'evidence-based' healthcare resources available on the internet, including peer-reviewed journals and 'eTextbooks'.
www.york.ac.uk/ Centre for Evidence Based Nursing, University of York.
www.york.ac.uk/inst/crd/ NHS Centre for Reviews and Dissemination.

Chapter 6

Quality in healthcare

NMC Standards of Proficiency

Contribute to public protection by creating and maintaining a safe environment of care through the use of quality assurance and risk management strategies.

Outcomes to be achieved for entry to the branch programme:
Contribute to the identification of actual and potential risks to patients, clients and their carers, to oneself and to others, and participate in measures to promote and ensure health and safety:

- recognise and report situations that are potentially unsafe for patients, clients, oneself and others.

Demonstrate a commitment to the need for continuing professional development and personal supervision activities in order to enhance knowledge, skills, values and attitudes needed for safe and effective nursing practice.

Outcomes to be achieved for entry to the branch programme:
Demonstrate responsibility for one's own learning through the development of a portfolio of practice and recognise when further learning is required:

- begin to engage with, and interpret, the evidence base which underpins nursing practice.

Chapter aims

After reading this chapter, you will able to:

- discuss what is considered to be good quality nursing care;
- explain how good-quality care can be achieved and maintained;
- identify the aims of clinical audit and clinical governance in the pursuance of quality;
- understand the role of the National Institute for Health and Clinical Excellence (NICE), the Commission for Healthcare Audit and Inspection (CHAI) and the National Service Frameworks (NSFs);
- consider your own role and personal qualities in the maintenance of quality care provision within the limits of your own abilities.

Introduction

Throughout the late 1980s and most of 1990s the NHS began to adopt a philosophy of quality in healthcare and treatment that mirrored the world of business. It was synonymous at the time with the development of NHS Trusts and subsequent considerations for maintaining and working within budgets, meeting targets and the competitive culture of market forces. Healthcare workers became known as 'purchasers' and 'providers', and GPs were encouraged to adopt 'fundholder' status to enable them to purchase services for their patients from the 'providers', namely hospitals and consultants. The cost of treatments featured more prominently in the delivery of healthcare and the need to provide a good-quality service became an essential component of these reforms.

Quality is a term that is often used to describe something favourably. It represents a benchmark or standard against which the worth or value of something is measured, for example 'that was a quality performance' or 'that was a good-quality meal'. While we can often judge the quality of a service or product as being 'good' or 'excellent', so too can we judge it as 'poor' or 'substandard'.

Whenever we experience something we tend to make an assessment of the quality of that experience by measuring it against our own expectations, for example what we thought it would be like, and then evaluating it in terms of how well it met the various criteria we used. Alternatively, there may be minimum standards laid down either in law or at a local level (e.g. health and safety, food hygiene) that subsequently guide our expectations and inform our individual assessment of the quality of the experience as we compare and contrast standards.

Judgements about quality are therefore based on how well the experience meets the expectation and whether or not it is fit for purpose. For example, if a service claims that it will achieve a certain standard, when that service is accessed, how well does it actually satisfy that claim? If certain requirements are laid down as expectations of the quality of a service, then the ongoing measurement of quality assurance is achieved by how well that service continues to meet the stated criteria. In this way minimum, acceptable standards of quality are achieved, along with the introduction of various drivers and incentives that are designed to gradually improve quality performance.

However, Ford and Walsh (1995) urge nurses to guard against simplistic definitions of quality as there is no objective and unique definition. They suggest that, because of its essentially subjective nature, quality can mean different things to different people.

In your own CFP your individual performance in practice as a student of nursing is measured against numerous criteria that identify the expectations that the nursing profession has regarding your progression and development at this stage. Periodic assessment of your work by qualified practitioners, measured against these criteria, provides an indication of your performance and acts as a guide to maintaining and improving your own personal standards, thereby contributing to the overall quality of care delivered to the patient. These expectations continue to ensure quality performance from students into the branch programme and beyond after your qualification as a registered nurse, where they are laid down locally in the form of job descriptions and professionally in the *Code of Professional Conduct* by the NMC (2008).

Whenever we access healthcare services, for whatever reason, all of us expect to receive good-quality treatment. Irrespective of how ill a person is, the provision of a good-quality service is central to the healthcare experience. Like so many other aspects of everyday life, whether it is in education, politics or even at our local supermarket, we expect a quality service and healthcare is no different.

Activity 6.1

Imagine that you have booked into a restaurant for a meal to celebrate an important occasion. Make a list of the various things that you would take into account when judging the quality of the meal.

A brief outline of what you might include on your list is at the end of the chapter.

Just as the quality of a meal in a restaurant can be judged by a number of different criteria, so too can the quality of healthcare.

Activity 6.2

You have been admitted to hospital for a minor operation. Although the procedure is routine and you will be going home later in the day, you are nonetheless a little anxious. What criteria will you use to judge the quality of the healthcare you will receive before and after your operation?

A brief outline of what you might include on your list is at the end of the chapter.

For Edwards (2005) the actual design of healthcare buildings comes into the quality equation. This could include a number of quality indicators, such as the available levels of technology, equipment, space, access, heating and toilet facilities. Any reduction or loss of these factors can affect the quality of the service provided or, as Edwards puts it, *will continue to disappoint and wear out the patience of those who pay the bills*. For this reason, since March 2005 the Commission for Healthcare Audit and Inspection (CHAI) undertakes an 'annual health check' of the NHS and Independent Care Providers in order to monitor and improve quality in service.

Commission for Healthcare Audit and Inspection

In April 2004, the Commission for Healthcare Audit and Inspection (CHAI; sometimes referred to as the Healthcare Commission) took over the role of the Commission for Health Improvement (CHI), which in turn was created by the Health and Social Care Act of 2003. The aim of CHAI (2005) is to promote improvement in the quality of NHS and independent healthcare by:

- safeguarding patients and promoting continuous improvement in healthcare services for patients, the public and carers;
- promoting the rights of everyone to have access to healthcare services and the opportunity to improve their health;

- being independent, open and fair in decision making and the consultative process;
- reviewing complaints about the NHS that have not been resolved.

The Commission intends to achieve its goals through a process of *inspecting*, *informing* and *improving* healthcare services in England and Wales. The *inspection* of health services involves the assessment of performance in the NHS as well as the registering and inspecting of individuals and organisations in the independent sector. The Commission intends to *inform* the public and patients of their findings through an annual rating system for NHS Trusts and an annual report on the state of healthcare to Parliament that will enable the public to then make informed decisions about healthcare. The *improvement* of services will be achieved through the dissemination of information, the assessment of performance and independent reviews, and investigations into complaints and serious failings. Annual health checks on NHS Trusts will monitor for safety, cost and clinical effectiveness, governance, patient-focused services, accessibility, responsive care and treatment, the care environment and public health.

Most recently, in September 2007, CHAI published a report entitled *Caring for Dignity*, which highlighted continuing concerns over the standards of care for older people in England and Wales. In particular, issues relating to privacy, single-sex wards, nutrition, communication and care of patients with dementia were raised as priorities. In addition, there are still concerns over the quality of care for older people from different ethnic groups, those at the ends of their lives and those living with disabilities. This report in essence assesses progress by NHS Trusts and the independent sector towards achieving the various goals set out in the *NSF for Older People* (DH, 2001a). This way, quality of service delivery is monitored for older people and recommendations for improvement are highlighted with deadlines for action approved.

Activity 6.3

Why do you think that older people highlighted the importance of single-sex wards as a measure of quality in healthcare?

An outline answer is provided at the end of the chapter.

It is worth considering the possible effect that ageism (Standard 1 of the NSF) might have on the provision of quality care for older people. Ageism is defined by Butler (1975) as 'discrimination against people because they are old'. Although, clearly, it is not the only explanation for the poor quality of service sometimes experienced by this client group, ageism is nonetheless a difficult and unacceptable aspect of healthcare in the twenty-first century that requires urgent attention. Ageism can be manifest in many processes, including using age as a criterion for deciding whether to treat a person or not. In addition to this, healthcare workers who possess inappropriate attitudes to their work with older people are more likely to provide a poor-quality service that fails to meet the needs of the client.

Another possible way of measuring quality is to compare and contrast the performances of individual Trusts and make this information public, so that people can judge for themselves the standards of healthcare across England and Wales. The idea for this type of quality comparison across hospitals originated in the USA and, in 1998, the first NHS league tables on safety and quality were published by the government in order to inform the public of places where standards were high, measuring performance criteria such as outpatient referral and appointment waiting times and length of hospital admissions for various conditions. However, more controversial measuring criteria, such as surgeon death rates for cardiac surgery, have led to considerable debate over the worth of such data to the general public, with claims that some pioneering surgeons are being disadvantaged. That said, there is emerging evidence that the recent reduction in cardiac death rates in parts of England is possibly attributable to the publication of such information.

Activity 6.4

In the mid-nineteenth century Florence Nightingale once remarked that *Hospitals should do the sick no harm.* What do you think she meant by this statement?

A brief outline answer is provided at the end of the chapter.

Clinical governance and National Service Frameworks

In 1999, the NHS Executive published a Health Service Circular entitled *Clinical Governance in the New NHS*, which detailed the government's intentions to improve quality and fair access within the service in line with their drive to modernise healthcare provision. The document built on the publication *A First Class Service: Quality in the new NHS* (DH, 1998b), with the intention to provide guidance on the implementation of a framework, within which local organisations could work to improve and assure the quality of services for patients.

The main aims of the initiative were to develop clear national standards for services and treatments through so-called National Service Frameworks (NSFs) and the creation of a new National Institute for Health and Clinical Excellence (NICE), along with a Commission for Health Improvement (CHI) to monitor progress. In addition, there was a commitment to modernising professional self-regulation and extended lifelong learning so that professionals can make best use of current evidence to inform their practice. A national survey of patient and user experience was undertaken to provide insights into the public perception of the health service.

The NHS was founded in 1948. It is a huge and complex organisation delivering healthcare in a variety of settings across the UK, ranging from large district hospitals, to those in the community and into people's homes. Within the NHS there are numerous HCPs who all work in the pursuit of clinical excellence and the delivery of high-quality care and treatment.

Activity 6.5

- Make a list of the various healthcare professionals (HCPs) who work within the NHS.
- Do you see any problems regarding communication between HCPs?

A brief outline answer is provided at the end of the chapter.

In *The NHS Plan* (2000) the DH describes the NHS as being a *1940s service operating in the 21st Century*. This implies that there is a perception that there are old-fashioned ways of working in the NHS that require modernising and changing to meet the needs of patients in today's world. By changing people's roles and ways of working within the organisation the intention is to improve quality and receptiveness to need. Clinical governance is seen as the framework for achieving this by *changing organisational culture* away from a *culture of blame* to one of learning so that quality infuses all aspects of the organisation's work (DH, 2000).

Key areas for change through clinical governance have been highlighted as:

- a new culture in NHS organisation;
- reducing inequity and variability;
- involving users and carers;
- sharing of good practice;
- detecting and dealing with poor performance and adverse events.

In order for clinical governance to be successful the government initiatives have been aimed at promoting a more open and participative culture within the NHS that values the sharing of education, research and good practice.

How might this improve quality? The sharing of good practice between professionals encourages more good practice to take place. Educating one another about latest developments and current research findings helps with this process by keeping people up to date. The breaking down of barriers between professional groups is seen as a hallmark of an organisation in which quality is likely to thrive; thus the flattening of hierarchies within the NHS is to be encouraged so that the old-fashioned demarcations between staff no longer exist (DH, 2000).

Over the years, since its inception, there have been growing concerns that the NHS has not fulfilled its founding principles – in particular that it should be 'egalitarian', i.e. treat people equally. Successive reports (Acheson, 1998; Black, 1980, cited in Townsend et al., 1992) have shown that unjustifiable variations in the healthcare experiences of various sectors of society have occurred in relation to the quality of services provided in different areas. This includes access to healthcare services as well as the overall outcomes and appropriateness of interventions. As a result of these concerns, and in order to standardise service provision throughout the NHS, a series of National Service Frameworks (NSFs) have been developed.

Activity 6.6

Make a list of the various NSFs that you are aware of. Visit the DH website at www.dh.gov.uk to check your list and make a note of the ones you missed.

As you will be checking your list on the website, there is no outline answer at the end of the chapter.

As you will see when completing Activity 6.6, NSFs have been developed over the past ten years or so for a variety of conditions with the aim to improve and standardise the care and treatment of people across the UK. In addition to this, various protocols for care delivery have been developed: these are often known as integrated care pathways (ICPs) and are designed to ensure that acceptable standards of both nursing and medical treatment are achieved. Many ICPs are now in operation, including those for Stroke Illness and Myocardial Infarction, and also for surgical interventions such as Total Hip Replacement and Transurethral Prostatectomy. ICPs complement both the NSFs and clinical governance.

There are other initiatives to improve standards in healthcare, such as the Essence of Care (EOC) benchmarking system (DH, 2001b), which not only provides healthcare practitioners with a series of indicators for best practice but also encourages the development of plans for addressing poor practice.

The specific areas of care currently targeted through EOC are:

- principles of self-care;
- personal and oral hygiene;
- nutrition;
- communication;
- continence and bladder and bowel care;
- pressure ulcers;
- safety of clients with mental health needs;
- record keeping;
- privacy and dignity;
- health promotion;
- care environment.

The government has also set up NICE to advise on the cost of various treatments for the NHS. NICE consists of a panel of experts who make decisions about various treatments based on the perceived longer-term benefits versus the cost implications. Some very difficult decisions have to be made about the economy of healthcare in the NHS as it does not have finite resources, meaning it cannot fund all treatments and interventions for all people. The role of NICE, although advisory, is nonetheless influential and respected. It helps to ensure quality provision for the majority by limiting expenditure on costly and sometimes unproven interventions. It makes informed, if at times seen as unpopular, decisions about healthcare provision. There will be more on this subject later in the chapter.

Clinical audit and quality assurance

One way of assessing the ongoing quality of service provision and to ensure that basic minimum standards are maintained is to undertake annual clinical audit. Audit processes involve selecting and reviewing certain activities within healthcare practice and then measuring the annual performance against various criteria to assess the standard. A standard is a measure of expectation, something to aspire to, a guideline for good or minimum best practice. Standards can be used to judge the worth or effectiveness of something or someone in a given situation. They apply to all of us in most aspects of everyday life and are essentially designed to guide human behaviour in such a way that is acceptable to the majority of people. In this respect, standards are derived from various sources, most importantly in law, employment and through religious and moral codes. Some of the earliest standards that we learn in life are passed down through the family network from our parents and can be later reinforced by the Church and in education, a process that is termed primary and secondary 'socialisation' by the discipline of Sociology. More recently, the media has played an increasing role in the reinforcement of moral standards within society by clearly portraying what is 'good' and 'bad' human behaviour.

In the world of work, employers exact standards of expectation and behaviour on their employees through the use of written contracts and job descriptions. This is turn is reinforced with the use of disciplinary procedures to address unacceptable behaviour in the workplace. In your role as a student of nursing, you will find that there are clearly defined standards of professional behaviour and proficiency that you are expected to achieve at various stages of your course. Some of these are highlighted at the start of this chapter, for instance. These standards are laid down by your university, the various NHS Trusts in which you will work and by the governing body for nurses and midwives, the NMC. In order to achieve a given standard, a number of benchmarks or criteria are defined to act as a guide or steps towards achieving a goal. You will encounter these in the various modules that you undertake in the CFP and the Branch Programme, as well as in the practice documents that will be used to assess your performance in the clinical area.

As previously mentioned, a good way of assuring the ongoing provision of acceptable standards and good quality care in nursing is through the use of clinical audit. Key areas that we shall concentrate on are record keeping and patient satisfaction levels.

Activity 6.7

Make a list of the various standards you would expect when reading a handwritten nursing report that documents the progression of a patient's care and treatment for a shift. Remember that, until computerised records of patient progress become more accepted and widespread in healthcare practice, written records will continue to be an important means of communication between HCPs.

A brief outline answer is provided at the end of the chapter.

Record keeping is just one way of measuring quality assurance through clinical audit. It is a valuable tool for ensuring that HCPs maintain good standards of written communication in their work, reducing ambiguity and confusion wherever possible. However, as you can appreciate, maintaining good-quality written records is an ongoing challenge that requires at least annual monitoring.

Another approach to clinical audit and ongoing quality assurance is to consult with the consumers of the service – the patients. This is at the very heart of the government reform agenda, with a commitment to empower and listen to patients as detailed in the NHS Improvement Plan (DH, 2004). What better way could there be of gaining insights into how well the service provision matches expectation than to ask the very people who access it? As a result this has become a frequently used measure of the quality of care provision. However, measuring patient satisfaction levels can be problematic, especially when deciding upon the approach to use and the timing. In Activity 6.2 you personally made an assessment of the quality of care you expected during a brief period in hospital for a minor operation, but what happens if you are dissatisfied with your experience of healthcare? Who do you complain to?

Various attempts to measure patient satisfaction have been introduced by NHS Trusts across England and Wales in order to inform clinical audit. The difficulties that are often faced by auditors include the actual understanding of what constitutes 'satisfaction' and the method by which it should be measured. How do we know when someone is satisfied with the care and treatment they have received: do they say so, or do they leave gifts, write a letter or send a card explaining their satisfaction perhaps?

Patient satisfaction, while recognised as an important means of gaining information about the service, is nonetheless notoriously difficult to measure as it is fraught with potential biases. People are less likely to complain about a service if they are dependent upon it for treatment. Nobody wants to be viewed as unpopular or, worse still, a troublemaker. There will be more discussion on the problems of measuring satisfaction levels in Chapter 8.

Personal qualities and professional behaviour

So far this chapter has concentrated on various aspects of quality in healthcare, ranging from clinical governance and audit to quality assurance. All of these terms should be more familiar to you now and you should have a better grasp of how quality can be measured and improved in the healthcare setting. Although the environment in which people work can sometimes affect the quality of nursing care delivered, it is mostly affected by the skills, knowledge and attitudes of the individuals working with the patient. While initiatives such as clinical audit can be used to monitor performance at a particular point in time, it is nevertheless the ongoing delivery of good-quality care and treatment throughout the 24-hour period, seven days a week, that people make judgements on. It is therefore the maintenance of high standards in one's own personal performance that contributes to the overall impression.

> ### Activity 6.8
>
> Take 20 minutes time out to think about your own professional values in your work. How will you ensure that your nursing standards are high and will contribute to the overall provision of good quality care? What skills, knowledge and attitudes will you need to achieve this? How will you maintain these standards throughout your nursing career?
>
> For possible answers to this question, see the text below.

The questions in Activity 6.8 are quite difficult to answer, but hopefully you will have identified the need to develop **competence** in your practice that will include not only the **manual practical skills** but also the **essential communication and listening skills** that will enable you to be sensitive and responsive to the needs of others in your care. You probably also thought of the importance of **knowing your own limitations** at this early stage in your career, by recognising **the need to refer to another more experienced and knowledgeable person**, such as your mentor, if you feel unable to act with confidence and competence at a given task. This is an essential part of your professional development and is an integral part of the provision of a good-quality and safe service to the public.

You may also have looked at aspects of **your own professional behaviour** and the various expectations that the NMC, your colleagues and the general public have of you. You might have identified **the need to be reliable** in your practice placement, and perhaps your appearance, your uniform and manner featured in your definition of **personal standards**. Indeed, members of the public expect to see someone who looks the part and is respectful and polite in their communications.

Perhaps you identified the importance of **teamwork**, **multidisciplinary working** and **good communication between professionals**. Even at this early stage in your nursing career you will play a very important part in the communication of your observations of patients to fellow HCPs. This may be verbally or under supervision in written form. Working as part of a team with a common goal is again an important part of your professional development and effective communication between HCPs improves the overall quality of healthcare provision.

You may have also thought of **the need to keep up to date with current practice** by **improving your knowledge base** and **finding out about things you have encountered**. The principle of lifelong learning is embodied in nursing and embraces evidence-based practice (EBP; see Chapter 5), whereby your actions can be justified through reference to the latest research findings. While learning from theory and practice will seem at its most intense during your three-year training period, continuing your education in the post-qualifying period is an important expectation of both the NMC and your employing authority. This ensures that you are knowledgeable and responsive to change in the healthcare arena.

National Institute for Health and Clinical Excellence

Earlier in the chapter we alluded to the concern that, in the past, there has been considerable variation in the levels of service provision within the NHS across the UK. This has led to inequity of access to healthcare for certain sectors of society that is largely dependent upon what is available in the area where you live – the so-called 'postcode lottery'. In 1999 the DH accepted that these variations existed and had earlier cited three main reasons for these problems (DH, 1998b):

- absence of clear standards of care for the NHS;
- lack of a coherent approach to assessment of good practice and what works best;
- slow and inconsistent uptake of effective treatments.

In response the DH set in motion a detailed long-term programme for quality improvement. This included establishing the National Institute for Health and Clinical Excellence (NICE) as an organisation that would provide national guidance on the promotion of good health and the prevention and treatment of ill health, as a means of minimising inequalities in healthcare. This was to be achieved by addressing the variations in practice and acting as a source of clinical guidance by advising on the cost-effectiveness of new medicines and other interventions within the NHS.

Three main areas of health have been targeted for action:

- **public health**: providing guidance on the promotion of good health and the prevention of ill health for those working in the NHS, for patients and their carers and wider society;
- **health technologies**: advising on the use of new medicines, treatments and procedures;
- **clinical practice**: providing guidance on appropriate treatment and care for those people with specific diseases and conditions.

In order to achieve its goals, NICE has developed a number of tools, such as cost templates, audit criteria and slide sets, to help facilitate discussion with audiences affected by the recommendations. In short, NICE advises on best practice by using the evidence available for a variety of conditions and treatments, and by using their costing templates to assist local authorities to assess the impact of the guidance on local budgets.

Activity 6.9

- **What do you understand by the term 'cost-effectiveness?**
- **How might the notion of cost-effectiveness be applied in healthcare?**
- **How might the quality of healthcare be linked to the cost-effectiveness of treatments?**

There is a brief outline answer at the end of the chapter.

Cost-effectiveness analysis (CEA), as undertaken by NICE, is a process by which comparisons between the costs and health effects of particular interventions are assessed, in order to ascertain whether they are worth doing from an economic perspective – the so-called *health gain*. Where resources are limited, as in the NHS, decisions about the cost-effectiveness of treatments, in terms of perceived and actual benefits, are of paramount importance, otherwise there are serious financial implications. However, decisions about costing can become controversial and emotive, especially if they mean that certain drugs will not be available because of their expense to the NHS. All decisions about cost and treatment availability in the NHS should also consider the various ethical implications.

NICE decisions are not always that popular with the public and it might be difficult to see at times how they contribute to the ongoing provision of good-quality care if they limit access to some treatments that might save lives and that people think should be available on the NHS. However, by reducing the amount of expenditure on expensive treatments, it is argued that more funds are then made available to a wider audience who can benefit from better standards of care more generally across the UK. In ethical terms, this is referred to as the 'utilitarian' approach whereby the aim is to achieve *the greatest good for the greatest number* (Mill, 2001). However, there are criticisms of this philosophy in healthcare, in particular that the needs of minority groups may be overlooked and that no one person can predict what actual health gains will be achieved in the future.

You may not have considered that the cost of treatment and care could ultimately affect the quality of service provision, but in 1948, at its inception, the NHS was founded on four major principles (Seedhouse, 1994):

- it should meet all heath needs;
- everyone should receive the best care;
- it should be egalitarian;
- it should keep the costs of healthcare as low as possible.

However, commentators argue that principles two and four are incompatible, as receiving the best care might mean that costs have to increase, especially where current technologies are needed to maximise the health gain. Equally difficult is the notion that all healthcare needs should be met, as this again has the potential to incur the greatest cost. The notion of egalitarian care and treatment has also suffered, as inequity in service provision has been argued at length and demonstrated in differences in infant mortality rates and life expectancy for lower social class groups since the publication of the Black Report in 1980 (cited in Townsend et al., 1992).

Over time the founding principles have been tempered to accommodate the growing concerns over health service expenditure. For example, the word 'best' tends to have been superseded by 'quality service' and there has been a gradual realisation among politicians and healthcare economists alike that not 'all' health needs can be met because of costs. As a result, maintaining the quality of service provision in the NHS is ultimately reliant upon the cost-effectiveness of the interventions employed. Whereas the quality of face-to-face encounters can be measured in terms of information giving, speed of response and politeness, the actual overall quality of treatment is dependent upon whether it is affordable in the first place. Therefore, some treatments may still be limited because of cost. As the quality of a particular experience is largely a subjective judgement, possibly varying from person to person, the government uses very broad criteria for measuring the quality of NHS work: for example, waiting list reductions and increases in nurse and doctor recruitment numbers that are easily measurable, quantifiable and can be demonstrated as real evidence of improvement.

The role of the media in quality assurance

In recent years the media in the UK, that is newspapers, radio and television reporting, have consistently focused on the achievements of the NHS. Hardly a week goes by without there being some kind of report or statement concerning the quality of care and treatment provided (see Chapter 3 for more information on the media's influence in policy-making). The advent of the internet as a means of mass communication has heightened the scrutiny of all matters to do with health, and NHS performance is always a major political talking point. Unfortunately, while instances of good practice are occasionally reported upon, many of the stories covered often detail inadequacies in the system by highlighting shortfalls or even poor, unacceptable practice. The tendency to focus on negative occurrences can give a rather false impression of the overall picture of treatment in the NHS and might even affect people's confidence in the service. While, collectively, NHS Trusts will always aspire to the provision of good or excellent care and treatment, it is inevitable that, within such large organisations employing literally thousands of people, occasionally standards will be compromised. While clearly not desirable, it is simply a statement of fact, and the need to minimise such occurrences is of paramount importance.

Consider the potential impact of the following newspaper headlines on public confidence in the NHS. Do you think that these types of stories are helpful?

- *Hospital bug deaths 'scandalous'* (*Guardian*, October 2007).
- *NHS bugs 'due to poor leadership'* (*Guardian*, October 2007).
- *NHS: I found a used needle by his bed* (*Daily Telegraph*, November 2007).
- *Slapdash nursing care blamed for night falls* (*Times*, October 2007).
- *Inquiry launched into why hospitals allow the elderly to go hungry* (*Daily Mail*, September 2007).
- *Malnutrition of elderly patients 'still a big worry'* (*Yorkshire Post*, August 2007).

Not exactly good publicity is it? But, nevertheless, this is a reflection of the type of scrutiny that the NHS is under in the twenty-first century. In order to prevent such headlines from occurring, all healthcare workers need to ensure that they are delivering high-quality care and treatment to the public. The media has increasingly played a role in informing the public of problematic situations within the NHS, but you might ask how representative are their views and how accurate are the reports they produce? Sometimes sensationalist headlines can be misleading and generate undue fear and mistrust. Without question, there are problems of quality within certain sectors of the NHS that need addressing, just as there always have been, but is it any worse now than it was, say, 60 years ago? The incidence of HAIs and the concerns over the malnutrition of elderly people in hospitals are just two of the current topics of debate in the political, nursing and media arenas.

Activity 6.10

Why do you think instances of poor practice occur in the NHS? What could be the possible explanations for this? Talk with qualified nurses about standards in healthcare and see if they share some of your ideas.

A brief outline answer is provided at the end of the chapter.

Let's take two of the issues raised in the answer to Activity 6.10 and explore the validity of the claims, namely those of 'not having enough time' and 'poor leadership'. Time is often used in healthcare as a reason for not being able to do things – 'we simply do not have the time' – but is this a legitimate excuse for poor and sometimes neglectful care and treatment?

In health, time is something that drives us all. It motivates us to get up in the morning, to go to work and to come home again in the evening. We judge our daily activities by how much time we have to complete them. We have appointments, we go to meetings and we have to be in certain places by a certain time. Time gives structure and order to our days and nights; in short, it provides us with a purpose for action.

Nurses are very busy people. They work hard and sometimes feel that their efforts are not always recognised. Time in nursing practice is of the essence and shift work is the epitome of time consciousness. However, the notion of time in nursing is very closely related to that of task orientation, that is, getting the job done and the orderly completion of daily tasks. In the past nursing has been criticised for various ritualistic practices that have little meaning or evidence to support their execution (Walsh and Ford, 1992; Ford and Walsh, 1995). Examples of these actions include the ritualistic recording of physical observations, such as a person's temperature when it is not needed, and the prolonged and unnecessary pre-operative fasting schedules for surgical patients. it is argued that, while nurses spend time engaged in these rather outdated practices, they may well be overlooking more important activities in their work.

For example, a common explanation for the failure to help elderly patients at mealtimes is that nurses do not have enough time to sit down and do this, because there are more pressing issues to attend to. Again, you may ask if this is a legitimate excuse? Helping poorly people to eat is indeed a time-consuming activity and it can also take a great deal of patience and perseverance, requiring considerable personal investment and motivation to sometimes achieve only the minimum of success. But it is not just about time; it is about valuing the activity and appreciating its overall worth and benefit to the patient.

So it would seem that perhaps quality is more than time itself. A great deal of good-quality care and treatment is achieved across the NHS every day by extremely busy people because they care about what they are doing and they want to do it well. Therefore, the provision of good-quality care encompasses an attitude to work that still excels in difficult circumstances.

However, there are, of course, circumstances where environments and the nature of the work can conspire to become very stressful, and the demands are such that the nursing role is affected because people find it difficult to concentrate. This might be because of the sheer volume of work expected or through poor leadership from people who find it hard to express themselves. Where workload is excessive, coupled with shortages of staff, stress can build and lead to a so-called 'burnout' that compromises standards. In these instances the claims over lacking time will be entirely justified and there is a need for strong leadership and clinical supervision to improve the situation.

This leads into the second issue relating to 'poor leadership' within nursing. There have been many critics of leaders in nursing and the profession is often seen as subservient to the medical profession. Some of this criticism has come from within the nursing profession itself. There have been instances of nurses feeling distinctly disempowered in their roles, disillusioned and dispirited. There is currently a focus in both the media and political arena on improving the quality of healthcare, particularly in the hospital setting, where it is thought that, since the demise of the hospital-based Matron some 30 years ago, standards have gradually fallen. The assertion has been that there is a need for a figurehead in nursing, that is, someone who embodies a sense of discipline and pride in the work, in order to restore confidence. As a result of this concern and following public consultation and a commitment in *The NHS Plan* (DH, 2000), the current Labour government reintroduced a 'Modern' Matron to hospital wards in 2002. The return of the Matron was welcomed by the public and within the profession itself. The remit of the role is to be a *strong clinical leader with clear authority* making the fundamentals right by *leading by example* (DH, 2003a). Two main objectives of the Matron are to target hospital cleanliness and prevent HAIs.

It will be in the ensuing years that we will learn the level of success achieved by the Matron, but the need for strong leadership is clear. Good leaders are ones who make things happen – inspirational people who encourage others to work together and transform practice. A good leader is someone who communicates clearly, provides feedback and support to their team, maximises potential within individuals and is an active participant in the provision of good-quality care. This is all achieved without taking full control or being overly authoritarian in their style. Without leadership, groups can sometimes lose their identity and focus, or may become unsure of their goals, thereby compromising care standards that can become disorganised and fragmented. Hopefully, the reintroduction of Matrons will bring about change for the better.

It is likely that the role of the media in highlighting instances of poor practice in the NHS will have some impact on the roles of HCPs by reminding them of the need to maintain good standards. Ongoing quality assurance requires extra vigilance in the provision of good-quality care. The extent to which the media portrayal of the state of the NHS in twenty-first century Britain affects the quality of the service is uncertain, but undoubtedly it has some effect in shaping perceptions and impressions of the type of services available. However, there is a danger that too much negative reporting might gradually erode public confidence, so therefore a more balanced approach is needed to share information about successful outcomes as well as those requiring improvement.

C H A P T E R   S U M M A R Y

- The definition of quality remains elusive, as it is essentially a subjective opinion – an individual judgement of the worth of something that can differ from person to person.
- Many attempts have been made to measure quality outcomes in healthcare and, since the late 1990s, many different tools, benchmarks, targets and milestones have been set up by the government in order to raise standards and improve the quality of service provision in the NHS.
- From a nursing perspective, quality is about providing care that adequately meets the needs of the person receiving it.
- As a student of nursing, quality is about developing your own personal standards through the guidance and supervision of more experienced nurses. It is about learning good ways for doing things, and being efficient and effective in your interactions with the users of the service.
- Quality is about acquiring knowledge and using evidence-based practice (EBP) to act and communicate effectively.
- Good-quality nursing is about motivation, compassion, sensitivity and respect for yourself and others. As long as you can maintain sufficient energy and motivation to want to do a job well, you will continue to deliver good-quality care.

Activities: brief outline answers

6.1 Restaurant quality (page 109)

It's likely that your list contains some of the following criteria:

- reputation of the restaurant;
- extent and choice of menu;
- cost of food;
- attentiveness of the staff, and their competence and manner;
- cleanliness of the surroundings, such as the restaurant itself, the cutlery, plates and toilets;
- ambience, such as comfort, lighting, decor and heating;
- tastiness and presentation of the food and the amount.

6.2 Healthcare quality (page 109)

There may be some similarities to your expectations from the previous activity, such as the cleanliness and decor of the hospital and/or unit that you are admitted to, along with the politeness and attentiveness of the staff.

However, you may also be looking for:

- prompt attention;
- good, clear communication and explanations from HCPs that keep you informed;

- truthful and honest answers to your questions;
- respect;
- correct use of your name;
- effective management of your pain.

All of the above aspects relate to the experience of healthcare from a personal perspective and as such are generally referred to as the *qualitative* as opposed to the *quantitative* elements of the service. Many recent research studies have concentrated on the healthcare experience from the patient perspective and these have helped shape service provision by informing and improving the quality of care to meet individual needs. These studies have provided important insights into the healthcare experience from an individual perspective that will be explored in more detail in Chapter 8.

6.3 Single-sex wards (page 110)

It is probable that people were thinking of preserving their dignity in everyday life, especially when they are at their most vulnerable. For example, there are particular concerns over the use of communal toilet and washing facilities in healthcare settings. The use of toilets, especially in illness, can be embarrassing, difficult and sometimes painful. This, coupled with possibly ill-fitting doors and/or a lack of privacy, can be very upsetting. There are several instances of gender divisions in wider society where men and women have different roles, most notably in sport, but gender differences are particularly obvious in relation to toilet and changing room facilities in the public domain. Why, then, would these general rules and expectations learnt from our culture be seemingly ignored in healthcare, especially in relation to older people?

6.4 Hospitals should do the sick no harm (page 111)

It is likely that Nightingale was referring to not making the patient's condition any worse through making mistakes, or perhaps through neglect, or through the contraction of the problems of bedrest, such as chest infections or pressure ulcers. She may also, given her record on cleanliness, have been referring to the threat of hospital-acquired infections (HAIs).

All of these problems are to do with the quality of care provision, but can they always be guarded against?

6.5 Healthcare professionals (HCPs) (page 112)

Apart from the obvious doctors and nurses, you might also have included the following:

- physiotherapists;
- occupational therapists;
- chiropodists/podiatrists;
- pharmacists;

- radiologists;
- health visitors;
- midwives;
- social workers.

In addition, there are other staff who are integral to the smooth functioning of the NHS, such as porters, secretaries, ward clerks and receptionists. There are also various specialist nurses involved in the care of patients, such as those working in the community, or in stoma care, breast care and cardiac rehabilitation.

Given the vast number of practitioners operating within the NHS, there are clearly issues regarding communication between individuals. Should there be a breakdown in communication, this could ultimately affect the quality of care as messages fail to be relayed correctly and misinformation leads to unnecessary delays in service response.

6.7 Standards for handwritten reports (page 114)

Perhaps you used the following criteria.

- Is the record legible?
- Is it accurate?
- Can it be understood?
- Are there any confusing phrases or abbreviations being used?
- Are there any unnecessary subjective statements about the patient included?
- Would a patient be able to understand the record?
- Has it been signed and dated, and by whom?

You need to familiarise yourself with the NMC's guidance on record keeping, which identifies key minimum standards for nurses (NMC, 2002a).

6.9 Cost-effectiveness (page 117)

Cost-effectiveness generally refers to a notion that someone is getting 'value for money' inasmuch as what is purchased is firstly affordable, and then worth the amount being paid for it in terms of the outcomes and benefits gained. If something is inefficient or actually costing more than the benefits of receiving it, then the overall quality of the service is brought into question and may not be sustainable in the future. Achieving maximum efficiency for minimal cost is the epitome of cost-effectiveness.

6.10 Poor practice (page 120)

Together you might have cited a number of reasons, such as not having enough time, being short-staffed, lacking resources, being stressed, suffering burnout, poor-quality staff, lacking knowledge, poor leadership, ageism and rigid, institutional care.

Knowledge review

Now that you have worked through the chapter, how would you rate your knowledge of the following topics?

	Good	Adequate	Poor
1. Quality in healthcare			
2. Clinical governance			
3. Quality assurance			
4. Cost-effectiveness in healthcare			
5. Professional standards			

Further reading

Craig, JV and Smyth, RL (2002) *Evidence Based Practice Manual for Nurses*, 2nd edition. Cheltenham: Churchill Livingstone.

Dawes, M, Davies, PT, Seers, K and Snowball, R (2005) *Evidence Based Practice: A primer for health care professionals*, 2nd edition. Cheltenham: Churchill Livingstone.

Department of Health (DH) (2003) *Winning Ways: Working together to reduce health care associated infection in England*. London: HMSO.

Useful websites

www.dh.gov.uk Provides access to all the recent policy documents from the Department of Health, including the various National Service Frameworks and other drivers for quality improvement in the NHS.

www.healthcarecommission.org.uk Carries the Healthcare Commission's latest recommendations for clinical practice, most importantly their recent report on *Caring for Dignity*, which details the necessary steps to improve quality care for older people. The Commission is the independent watchdog for healthcare in England and promotes continuous improvement in the provision of NHS services.

www.nice.org.uk National Institute for Health and Clinical Excellence: an important website detailing the latest proposals and recommendations from NICE – the body that provides guidance on clinical issues in the pursuance of promoting good health and treating ill health.

www.nmc-uk.org The official website of the Nursing and Midwifery Council – the governing body for nurses and midwives. It explains the latest developments in professional regulations and, most importantly, you can gain access to various documents, such as the 2008 *Code of Professional Conduct* and guidelines for record keeping and maintaining confidentiality. In addition, the website offers advice on professional matters.

Chapter 7

The patient perspective

NMC Standards of Proficiency continued

Formulate and document a plan of nursing care, where possible, in partnership with patients, clients, their carers and family and friends, within a framework of informed consent.

Outcomes to be achieved for entry to the branch programme:
Contribute to the planning of nursing care, involving patients and clients and, where possible, their carers; demonstrating an understanding of helping patients and clients to make informed decisions:

- participate in the negotiation and agreement of the care plan with the patient or client and with their carer, family or friends, as appropriate, under the supervision of a registered nurse;
- inform patients and clients about intended nursing actions, respecting their right to participate in decisions about their care.

Chapter aims

After reading this chapter, you will able to:

- appreciate the valuable contribution that patients and clients can make to their own care provision;
- realise how one's own values and attitudes might affect relationships with others;
- respect the autonomy of others in the decision making process;
- recognise the contribution of the Expert Patient Programme to the delivery of care and treatment for people with LTCs;
- understand patient anxiety and discuss strategies to reduce it.

Introduction

Most of us at some point in our lifetime will require the services of the medical profession, either from a personal perspective or perhaps for a family member. If the doctor examining you goes on to diagnose a specific problem and subsequently prescribes a course of treatment, then you enter into a professional relationship in which you are often viewed as a 'patient'. Although many other terms such as 'consumer', 'service user' and 'client' have been used interchangeably in recent years, reflecting the changing status and expectations of people accessing the health service, the term 'patient' nevertheless retains its dominance in everyday use in healthcare settings, particularly in adult nursing, and continues to feature prominently in the healthcare literature of the early twenty-first century. However, the notion of being labelled a patient has several connotations that have led some commentators to question its worth and relevance, as it is a term that is thought to reflect dependency, a lack of knowledge and power, and a degree of subservience to the medical profession, subjecting people to so-called 'paternalism'.

Activity 7.1

During your clinical placements in the CFP you will meet numerous patients in various healthcare settings. Think for a moment what the word 'patient' means to you and what expectations you might have of someone who is in this role. Make a list of your ideas and consider where these have come from.

A brief outline answer is provided at the end of the chapter.

The various expectations you will probably have thought about during Activity 7.1 reflect the traditional nurse–doctor–patient relationship that emerged during the inception of the NHS and the ensuing years. In 1951, Talcott Parsons, a social scientist, coined the phrase the 'sick role' to describe a set of expectations that guide patient behaviour. They are repeated below and were at the time very influential in shaping the HCP's view of patients and their use of the service. As you read through them, consider if they are still applicable to the twenty-first century. Are there any similarities in your own assessment of patients and that of Parsons some 60 years earlier?

According to Parsons (1951) in accepting the 'sick role' the patient gains two benefits, but at the same time is expected to fulfil two obligations:

Benefits
- The patient is temporarily excused his or her normal role.
- The patient is not responsible for his or her illness.

Obligations
- The patient must want to get well.
- The patient must cooperate with technically competent help.

Clearly, some of these expectations of the role of the patient have changed over time, although others still remain. While one of the benefits, 'being excused from your normal role', is still valid, the second concerning responsibility has started to change. Whereas most patients are still not directly held responsible for their illnesses, there is nevertheless a growing trend in healthcare to identify certain people, such as intravenous drug users, alcoholics, the morbidly obese and smokers, as somehow contributing to their own health problems. Again, it could be asked if this is a fair and just way of viewing poorly people, without knowing the full circumstances of their situation.

As regards obligations, there may be occasions when the patient does not want to get better, perhaps because of depression, infirmity or chronic unresolved pain that has affected their motivation to live. Alternatively, it might be the case that there is actually no cure for their condition and as a result it has become an integral part of their everyday lives.

The notion of cooperation with technically competent help is clearly an ongoing expectation of the patient role that is still applicable in contemporary healthcare practice; however, on occasions and for whatever reason, some people do not want to cooperate with or adhere to the recommendations of HCPs. Rather than labelling people as 'uncooperative' and 'difficult', it is important to be flexible in our approach to nursing patients and attempt to understand the possible reasons behind their non-adherence to medical regimens and advice.

Challenging paternalism

Clearly some of the older expectations of patient behaviour have started to change over time as people come to expect more information from those working in the NHS and to be consulted much more in the decision-making process concerning treatment and care. As previously suggested, critics of Parsons' perceptions of the so-called 'sick role' claim that this has led to a 'paternalistic' approach to healthcare, whereby the HCP, most often the doctor or nurse, is seen as an 'expert' and consequently takes over full responsibility for treatment of the patient and may even make decisions about care without involving the very person it affects. This 'doctor knows best' philosophy to healthcare practice is seen as a rather old-fashioned way of working in the NHS in the twenty-first century (DH, 2000) and the commitment to changing this approach is one of the driving forces behind the government's agenda for reform, which encourages greater patient involvement through a process of empowering and listening to the people who use the service (DH, 2004). In addition, with the advent of the internet and its many avenues of information gathering has emerged a new generation of enquiring individuals who can ask some searching questions. However, it is well worth remembering that not all information on the web is accurate or reliable and sometimes misconceptions need challenging.

The gradual shift of power from the professional to the service-user has meant that relationships are changing in order to reflect this new collaboration. This has involved much greater consultation with patients in order to understand their particular perspective, listening to their experiences and discussing their preferences by giving and expanding patient choice. Recent initiatives that have increased user involvement in treatment and care decisions include the Expert Patient Programme (DH, 2001d), the NHS Improvement Plan (DH, 2004), the Dignity in Care Campaign (DH, 2006f) and consultation with various patient groups such as the Patients Association (PA) and the Long Term Conditions Alliance (LTCA).

Scenario from practice

During the CFP you will nurse a number of people who are suffering from long-term conditions (LTCs). These are conditions that can last for many years, sometimes decades, as the person learns to cope with and adapt their lives to the various limitations or challenges they face. Some examples of LTCs include rheumatoid arthritis, heart disease, asthma, stroke illness and diabetes

Scenario from practice continued

mellitus. The DH (2005a) has also developed an NSF for long-term neurological conditions to standardise and improve care and treatment for this client group.

Imagine that you are visiting someone in their own home who has endured a chronic illness for over 20 years. Consider what benefits there would be in consulting with this person over their care needs. What valuable insights into their condition and strategies they use to manage their activities of living might be revealed? Listening to the patient's perspective can often reveal important pieces of information that can complement and enhance the plan of care such as:

- **how they manage their pain;**
- **what they use to mobilise;**
- **where they like to sit or lie;**
- **how they dress themselves and what aids to daily living they use;**
- **how they feel about their condition, their fears, anxieties and needs;**
- **what specific problems they and their carers face.**

Without this information the plan of care is incomplete as it lacks the necessary needs and wants of the individual. Not consulting with, or listening to, the patient can lead to several problems, including the risk of paternalism that the patient could find insulting, patronising and disrespectful. So much can be learnt from just taking the time to sit and listen to the patient perspective.

Improving patient satisfaction

Apart from listening to the individual's perspective on their own care and treatment, there are several other ways of gaining information from the public about what kind of service they would like. For example, patient surveys are often used as a means of gathering views and opinions, and there is a growing body of nursing research that examines the experiences of people who are living with conditions in order to provide important insights that can enhance future healthcare delivery.

Following growing concerns over the dignity in care for older people in the UK, the DH launched The Dignity in Care Campaign to *stimulate a national debate around dignity in care and create a care system where there is zero tolerance of abuse and disrespect of older people* (DH, 2006f). This is a good example of how consultation with the public through an online survey can be used to inform, shape and improve services. In this particular instance (DH, 2006f) over 400 people took part, commenting on their own experiences of care and subsequently identifying a number of characteristics of dignity that included:

- putting the individual receiving care at the centre of things, asking what their specific wants and needs are and how they want services to be provided;
- being patient;
- not patronising the person;

- helping people feel they can rest and relax in a safe environment;
- making sure people are not left in pain;
- respecting basic human rights, such as giving privacy and encouraging independence;
- taking into account people's cultural and religious needs.

As you can see, this is quite a comprehensive list and might actually contain certain aspects of dignity that some HCPs have not considered. Having these various items identified by actual users of the health service can help to inform all care workers who work with vulnerable elderly people in order to improve standards of dignity in care. Of course it will be necessary to conduct a review of healthcare provision for older people in the future in order to ascertain if any improvement has occurred as a result of these recommendations. For this reason the government often builds milestones or deadlines into their documentation as dates for reviewing progress towards improvement.

The nursing literature in recent years has contained some very good quality research studies on the experience of healthcare from a wide variety of personal perspectives. These are called qualitative studies (see Chapter 5 for a fuller discussion of this concept), because they examine the quality, not quantity, of healthcare outcomes and provide healthcare workers with important insights into the personal worlds of patients and how they perceive their conditions, their treatment and those around them. Invaluable information about the actual quality, good or bad, of healthcare provision can be gleaned from these articles, including the actions of nurses and doctors in the empowerment of others. This is why keeping up to date with current thinking and perspectives is such an integral part of your professional practice. For example, a study by Attree (2001), involving consultation with patients and their relatives, revealed information concerning their experiences and perspectives on what they described as 'good-quality care' and 'not so good-quality' care. The findings were as follows.

Good-quality care
- Individualised.
- Patient-focused and related to need.
- Humanistic.
- Caring staff who demonstrated 'involvement', 'commitment' and 'concern'.
- Respect for individuals' rights, dignity and privacy.
- Patients involved in decisions.

All of these positive statements reflect a type of care provision that at its heart fundamentally respects patients as people. From listening to patient perceptions of care we can identify the types of qualities, skills, knowledge and attitudes that nurses need to demonstrate effectively in their role.

Not so good-quality care
- Routine.
- Unrelated to need.
- Impersonal.

- Distant staff who do not know or involve patients.
- Unwillingness to help.
- Lacking respect.
- Limited communication.

All of these more negative statements about instances of care clearly reflect a particular attitude to work that is not conducive to individualised care, whereby people's own individual needs are not properly assessed or met. Here, it seems that the patient's experiences of healthcare leave a lot to be desired. Both the research study by Attree (2001) and the findings of the Dignity in Care Campaign (DH, 2006f) complement one another inasmuch as they illustrate a desire among the general public to receive healthcare and treatment that not only respects them as individuals but also preserves their dignity at a vulnerable time.

Further insights are provided by Webb and Hope (1995), who found that patients preferred a 'warm, friendly style of nursing' – one that embraced the important nursing activities such as 'listening to patients' worries', 'teaching them about their conditions' and 'relieving pain'. Interestingly, this study also identified a dislike of the use of first names, especially for older people. By consulting with their client group nurses can begin to tailor the service they provide to meet more effectively the needs of individuals in their care.

As discussed in Chapter 6, another way of obtaining information from patients concerning how they feel about the quality of the service they have received is through the use of satisfaction surveys. However, Walsh and Walsh (1999) suggest that patient satisfaction ratings often lack sensitivity, consistently achieving high scores. They also argue that they fail to isolate the specific nursing component from the whole healthcare experience. There are also problems with the timing of the surveys – when should they be done? Should they be carried out while the patient is in hospital, or perhaps just prior to discharge, or what about retrospectively when they are at home some days later?

Some examples of the types of questions asked in satisfaction surveys are as follows.

- Do staff use your preferred name? *Always/Sometimes/Never*
- Do doctors introduce themselves to you? *Always/Sometimes/Never*
- Do doctors explain what they are doing when examining you? *Always/Sometimes/Never*
- How easy is it to ask staff questions about your care? *Easy/Quite easy/Difficult*
- If you ring for assistance, how quickly do nurses respond? *Very quickly/Quickly enough/Too slowly*
- Do staff respect your wishes about how you want to be cared for? *Always/Sometimes/Never*
- Do nurses explain what they are doing while treating you? *Always/Sometimes/Never*

As you can see, all of the questions are specifically designed so that the patient can express an opinion on the care they are receiving; this can then be used by auditors to provide feedback to HCPs on the quality of service they are providing. Patients are usually given choices to respond to, such as the categories *Very quickly/Quickly enough/Too slowly* for the 'request for assistance' question. This way a general impression of the speed of response rate can be gleaned from reviewing the questionnaires. Providing categories to choose your answer from enables the collection of statistical evidence that can then be presented to staff in order to advise them either on the possible need for change or to reinforce good practices. However, as previously mentioned, questionnaires of this type do have limitations and sometimes patients consistently rate their experiences highly, which can somewhat skew the findings.

Activity 7.2

Having read the above on satisfaction surveys, answer the following question.

• Why do you think that some patients rate their care very highly?

There is a brief outline answer at the end of the chapter.

Expert Patient Programme

'My patients understand their condition better than I do' is an often used quote from doctors to describe how they feel when working with people with LTCs (chronic illnesses). But what do you think doctors mean by this statement? In what respect could patients know more than their doctors? Clearly, there is a growing acknowledgement in healthcare that someone who has lived for many years with a chronic medical condition will have developed various ways of coping and has important insights into their own illness that may not be known to the HCP. As a result of this recognition, there has been a considerable drive to develop what is termed the Expert Patient Programme (EPP) in order to harness and improve this expertise among those patients who are affected by LTCs.

Unfortunately, there are many instances of HCPs failing to listen adequately to their patients and equally failing to effectively treat and relieve some of the distressing effects of LTCs, such as pain and fatigue. This has led to some people with LTCs feeling abandoned by the NHS. It is very important to remember that the patient is the only person who truly knows what it is like to live with the condition. The EPP is designed to move away from the 'doing to' model of care and treatment through the empowerment of the patient to make decisions about their own care. The old-fashioned model of 'doctor knows best', which for so long induced passivity and dependence, could easily sap patients' self-confidence and undermine them, thus leading to stress and depression (LTCA, 2006/7).

Activity 7.3

Chronic pain, that is, pain that never seems to go away, is probably the leading cause of depression for people with LTCs. Chronic, unresolved pain can affect a person's concentration, emotions and willingness to move and carry out their daily activities. This is turn can heighten the feelings of depression, such as low mood, sadness, lack of motivation and lack of interest in things around them. In turn, if a person is still of working age, then pain of this type can affect employment prospects and willingness to work.

Think of a patient you have recently nursed who complained of chronic pain. How did he or she describe the pain and what did the nurse or doctor do to relieve the problem?

There is a brief outline answer at the end of the chapter.

The DH (2001d) estimates that, at any one time, as many as 17.5 million adults are living with chronic diseases in the UK, with older people suffering more. The implication is that, because collectively we have benefited from better healthcare and living conditions throughout the twentieth century, the resulting increase in longevity brings with it the increased risk of chronic illness for some people. So-called LTCs, because they affect people for a long and unspecified period of time, cannot be cured but they can be managed through the use of medication and other therapies.

Unfortunately, given the vast number of people with LTCs, the costs of treatment to the NHS are very high and some people with such conditions also suffer the paradox of inequalities in health service provision, depending on where they live and what is available to them in their locality.

The EPP's foundations were laid down in the DH's (1999a) Health Strategy White Paper, *Saving Lives: Our healthier nation*, with the setting up of an Expert Patient Task Force, and reaffirmed a year later in *The NHS Plan* (DH, 2000).

The general aims of the EPP (DH, 2001d) are to build the patient's confidence, knowledge and motivation so that they can utilise their own skills and information in order to manage their condition more effectively. The programme is also about encouraging liaison with professional services to address some of the complicating factors of chronic illness, such as pain, stress and low self-esteem, and to develop strategies to improve coping skills. Emphasis throughout is on patient self-management and regaining control of individuals' lives.

In order to support the initiative, Expert Patient Trainers (EPTs), who are also living with LTCs, have been appointed to work with PCTs across the country to offer courses to the public on the self-management of conditions such as multiple sclerosis, diabetes mellitus, asthma, heart disease, arthritis, endometriosis and stroke. Thus, the EPP reflects the new emphasis on partnerships between HCPs and patients.

The vision of the EPP (DH, 2001d), if successful, will show that:

- more patients with chronic disease improve, remain stable or deteriorate more slowly;
- more patients can manage effectively specific aspects of their condition, such as pain, medication and complications;
- patients with chronic disease are less severely incapacitated by fatigue, low energy levels, sleep deprivation and the emotional aspects of the illness;
- patients with chronic disease are effective in accessing health and social care services and in gaining and retaining employment;
- patients are well informed about their condition and medication, feel empowered in their relationship with HCPs and have higher self-esteem;
- people with chronic disease contribute their skills and insights for further service improvements and act as advocates for others.

Activity 7.4

In addition to the EPP, the Long Term Conditions Alliance (LTCA), established in 1989, works to meet the needs of people with LTCs. It too has vision and mission statements that are worth considering:

Vision: A world where people affected by LTCs have control over their lives and can live them to the full.

Mission: To ensure people affected by LTCs have access to the services and support they need, and can be active participants in determining their care.

Are there any similarities between these statements and the overall aims of both the Department of Health and the Expert Patient Programme?

There is a brief outline answer at the end of the chapter.

It will be many years before we are in a position to ascertain the true effects of the EPP on patient self-management skills. However, some preliminary statistics have already been released by the DH to demonstrate that the EPP is beginning to have some effect for individuals 4–6 months after attending the course, with the need for GP consultations, Outpatient Department visits and A & E visits all reduced, perhaps indicating an increased level of self-management and problem solving.

However, it remains to be seen how the EPP will reach out to those individuals who are affected by the inequalities of health service provision, and those who might be housebound, depressed because of their conditions, suffering with chronic pain and enduring long-term digestive problems (Hyde et al., 1999; LTCA, 2006/7).

Patient anxiety

The nature of illness and medical treatment is such that it can generate considerable anxiety in people.

Activity 7.5

What sort of things do you think might concern people when they are undergoing treatment and care in a hospital setting? Why might some people become anxious?

There is a brief outline answer at the end of the chapter.

In order to help reduce anxiety in hospitalised patients, nurses need to appreciate how some of the people they may be nursing are feeling. For example, this is especially important when the person is faced with the prospect of major, possibly disfiguring, surgery. The nurse can play an important part in building confidence and, if possible, helping people come to terms with the future. This can be invaluable in the post-operative period when patients may be gradually adjusting to changes in their appearance and bodily functions. However, despite the significance of this role, it is sometimes overlooked and undervalued (Jenkinson, 1996).

Activity 7.6

In order for you to begin to understand some of the issues surrounding anxiety, answer the following questions.

- **How would you recognise that someone was anxious?**
- **How might a nurse help to reduce anxiety in a patient?**

There are brief outline answers at the end of the chapter.

It is worth remembering that an overly anxious person may be more difficult to nurse because they might not listen to instructions and might misinterpret what is said to or asked of them, feel pain more intensely and suffer greater anticipatory anxiety that might make consent to procedures and their subsequent cooperation that much more difficult. People who are anxious or unsure of situations might also do unpredictable things and not adhere to the advice they are offered.

However, some people might have good reason for becoming anxious because of the actions of some doctors and nurses. Questioning the competence of someone who seems unsure of what they are doing can generate profound anxiety. At times patients can be quite vulnerable, especially if very poorly, and they have become reliant on the skills of the various HCPs around them. Misinformation concerning treatment regimens is a major source of concern; therefore, a nurse needs to be assured of their own level of knowledge and competence so as not to mislead patients when explaining things. Performing practical skills competently under supervision is an important part of your role as a student of nursing. However, it is important to try not to transfer your own anxiety about practical skills to the patient when at the bedside.

Developing appropriate communication skills, particularly those relating to listening and responding, helps to build not only your own confidence in stressful situations, but also that of the patient who then has faith in your abilities and trusts your actions and advice. Developing good communication skills is therefore an integral part of a competent nurse's role.

The difficult patient and the problem of labelling

In the course of their work nurses come into contact with people from a variety of backgrounds, each with his or her own individual experiences of life. This means that nurses are very likely to meet people from different cultures and find themselves caring for individuals who may have different values and lifestyles from their own (see Chapter 4 for further information). There may even be differences in the use of language between the professional and the patient, particularly concerning the use of words to describe parts of the body and their functions.

Social class has long been identified as a significant factor in determining the quality of the professional and patient interaction in healthcare. It is well recognised that many people who work in the health service tend to be middle class in origin and therefore may occasionally encounter difficulties when working with people from different backgrounds (Sheaff, 2005). This is a particular issue in the medical profession, where essentially middle-class, well-educated personnel can find themselves talking with patients from lower social groups about lifestyle issues of which they may have little knowledge or understanding, leading both parties to focus on different aspects (Mulcahy, 2003). Barriers such as language and failure to understand behaviours and ways of life could easily lead to labelling people as 'uncooperative' or 'difficult' and may even account for the differences in consultation times that have been noted between some doctors and certain sectors of society (Cartwright and O'Brien, 1976, cited in Sheaff, 2005). The various environmental and social determinants of health and illness, such as lifestyle, housing and occupation, need to be considered whenever treating or caring for someone.

From the previous section on anxiety you can now appreciate that, when people become ill and require treatment that may necessitate a period of hospitalisation, they can experience considerable anxiety that might on occasions alter their behaviour. Sometimes this behaviour may not match the expectations of what a 'good' patient should be like and, if repeated, might actually lead to the person being labelled as 'difficult' or being deemed to have acted in a deviant way. You might be surprised to learn that there are numerous instances in both nursing and medical literature of the term 'the difficult patient' being used. One of the earliest nursing studies into the phenomenon was by Felicity Stockwell (1972), whose influential work *The Unpopular Patient* identified certain types of people towards whom nurses developed unfavourable attitudes; these included individuals who were 'unpleasant', 'rude', 'demanding', 'attention seeking' and 'uncooperative'. Other studies have also identified a plethora of negative labels, including 'the non-compliant', 'the stubborn', 'the angry', 'the violent' and 'the drunk' or 'alcoholic' (Kelly and May, 1982). There is also the notion that, on occasions, there are inappropriate admissions to hospital, such as for those who 'self-harm' (Williams, 2007).

Nurses are in a privileged position, as the nature of their work means that they have access to considerable personal information about the various people in their care. This information can include patient diagnosis, the reasons for current admission, past medical history and even details on where the patient lives. Some of this sensitive information might trigger thoughts and feelings towards the patient even before they arrive. In the course of your duties as a nurse it is important to maintain confidentiality at all times and recognise that some of the value-laden labels attached to difficult patients have the potential for creating bias in your work.

From the list of patient types presented above we can see that certain people whom nurses encounter and, for whatever reason, find difficult to nurse can be labelled in a simplistic yet quite negative way, which then has the potential to affect the type of care and treatment they receive. From the patient's perspective, this is problematic and is referred to as *non-caring* by Carveth (1995). Non-caring actions can manifest themselves in nurses spending less time with unpopular patients or sometimes avoiding them altogether. You might question whether it is fair or ethical to spend more or less time with patients in your care.

Patient scenario

Imagine you are a patient in hospital who has been asking a lot of questions about your care and treatment because you want facts and clarification. However, unbeknown to you, nurses and doctors have labelled you as 'demanding and argumentative' because of the sometimes difficult questions you ask. How would you feel if you thought that nurses were now deliberately avoiding you or just spending the bare minimum of time in your company?

It is possible that you might feel angry, saddened, helpless, frustrated, bitter, puzzled, confused or even hurt. All of these emotions will further affect your behaviour and could make you even more demanding as you struggle to regain control over your situation.

It is interesting to think that, just because someone asks for information, they might be labelled so negatively, but it could be the nature of the questions being asked and the manner in which it is done that has affected the staff perceptions. While not condoning the actions of the staff in this scenario, it nonetheless offers a possible explanation for the difficulties arising.

Williams (2007) suggests that it is through the language nurses use, both verbal and non-verbal, especially during handover, that some of these negative messages about individual patients are conveyed. This information can then form impressions in people's minds before they even meet the patient in question. Another problem with using the 'difficult' label is that, once it has been applied and is then reinforced at handover or through nurse–doctor exchanges, there is a danger that the patient's subsequent behaviour will be interpreted in relation to the label and as a result they seem to behave just as expected. This illustrates how easily false beliefs about someone can become perceived as true simply through social interaction, a phenomenon that in educational psychology is referred to as the 'self-fulfilling prophecy' (Rosenthal and Jacobson, 1968).

Activity 7.7

While on your next clinical placement, listen to the words and phrases that are used to describe patients during the handover. What sort of impressions did you form in your mind of the patients you were going to nurse? Having met the people described, were the reports of their behaviour accurate or misleading?

A brief outline answer is provided at the end of the chapter.

For Kelly and May (1982) labelling in healthcare occurs as a consequence of the interaction between staff and patients. If the patient fails to meet the expectations of acceptable behaviour, they will be labelled accordingly. If a person says or does something that is inappropriate, unusual or offensive, then this can trigger negative feelings towards them. For this reason Johnson and Webb (1995) urge nurses to look beyond the individual circumstance and see how the context of care might be contributing to the difficulties. There may be a good number of other reasons why this patient is behaving in this way, including the lack of a harmonious environment, which is causing stress to all concerned (Macdonald, 2007). In situations like this, where staff are increasingly stressed, overstretched and working under great pressure, patients may pick up on these anxieties, which in turn affects their behaviour. A so-called 'demanding' patient may also be a very anxious one. Therefore, the key to resolving difficulties lies more in understanding the possible causes of the behaviour rather than rigid labelling that has the potential to disadvantage the patient.

Activity 7.8

Make a list of the qualities that a nurse will need in order to reduce the potential for bias in his or her interactions with patients.

There is a brief outline answer at the end of the chapter.

It is clearly in the best interests of all concerned to attempt to resolve conflict. This can be achieved in part by listening to and understanding the patient's perspective, even if their behaviour has already been labelled as 'difficult' or 'inappropriate'. Much of the blame for difficult behaviour in patients is often centred on the individual who is personally held responsible for the problems in the professional relationship. For some people this may be an accurate perception, but for many others the cause of their behaviour might be rooted in wider contextual issues that are threatening their well-being and safety. Often people are inappropriately labelled because of extreme anxiety, fear or poor coping mechanisms that lead them to behave in a 'difficult' way. A nurse can do a great deal to understand the situation, accurately perceive the patient's feelings and resolve the difficulties arising.

CHAPTER SUMMARY

- Without due consultation with the patient – the so-called patient perspective – the delivery of care and treatment is incomplete as it fails to take into consideration the needs of the very person being cared for.
- Healthcare provision at the beginning of the twenty-first century has at its heart a commitment to increasing patient autonomy, giving people choices and listening to the public perceptions of the NHS.
- The relationship between HCPs and patients is changing away from the old model of paternalism to a more person-centred approach.
- This new philosophy is reflected in the DH's commitment to NHS reform and the implementation of the EPP to drive forward the improvements in self-managed care for LTCs.
- At the centre of your role as a student of nursing is the practice of good communication skills, through which you can demonstrate respect and consideration for the patients in your care.
- Listening to patients' concerns and responding in a helpful, supportive and positive manner will help some people to develop the confidence they need to make decisions about their own conditions and treatment.
- In the course of your career as a nurse you will encounter many different people with differing healthcare needs. It is hoped that this chapter has provided you with some important insights into the type of skills you will need to develop in order to become a partner in care with the patients you meet.

Activities: brief outline answers

7.1 Meaning of the word 'patient' (page 128)

It is likely that your list will have included some of the following, and that you might expect a 'patient' to:

- be ill and needing treatment and care to get better;
- be cooperative and adhere to the various treatments prescribed;
- be polite;
- be respectful;
- listen to advice;
- want to get better.

7.2 Satisfaction surveys (page 133)

When patients rate their care very highly, there is always the possibility that their care is indeed very good and they are just reflecting this degree of satisfaction in their answers.

However, the validity of this type of assessment can be questioned, as sometimes people might not be as honest or as truthful as expected, especially if they suspect that the information they supply might be used against them in some way. Patients in hospital will always want to receive good care, so they might just be tempted to rate it as good, in order to keep the peace. Even though the questionnaires are always anonymous, to be too critical of a service might just be counterproductive.

Given the potential problems in both the interpretation and validity of patient satisfaction questionnaires, any findings should be treated with caution. It is perhaps the timing of the administration of the questionnaire that needs careful forethought and planning, so that patients do not feel threatened or pressurised into responding in a particular way.

7.3 Chronic pain (page 134)

People use a variety of words to describe their pain, such as 'stabbing', 'grinding', 'aching', 'discomfort', 'excruciating', 'agony', 'annoying'. Pain is a very subjective experience, and each of us uses differing words to describe a sensation that is real and upsetting. Pain also has different meanings for different people, making it a very complex phenomenon. For the person with chronic pain there can also be a sense of helplessness and/or hopelessness, when nothing seems to change the pain or make it go. It might also mean that a person cannot rest or sleep and this accentuates their low mood.

It is likely that the nurse or doctor would have listened to the patient and undertaken an assessment to ascertain the severity of the pain and then administered some form of analgesia. However, it is important to remember that some types of chronic pain are very difficult to treat with analgesia and that other forms of therapy may be necessary.

In either case, a detailed assessment of the patient needs to be done with the nurse or doctor and patient working in partnership to resolve this distressing aspect of some LTCs, such as arthritis. Again, consultation with the patient is vital in order to understand the meaning of pain for the person. Even if the pain cannot be completely relieved, at least having the opportunity to talk about it to someone who listens and shows compassion might help in some small way and reduce the feelings of helplessness and isolation that often accompany this type of pain.

7.4 LTC management (page 135)

Hopefully, you will have noticed that there really is a drive towards empowering patients and liberating them from the old ways of working in the NHS. The philosophy of increasing patient autonomy and choice is evident in both statements and reflects an ongoing commitment to improving the management of LTCs for the millions of people who suffer from them.

7.5 Anxiety (page 136)

Your answer should have identified a good number of factors, such as:

- fear of the unknown;
- uncertainty;
- fear of death;
- unresolved pain;
- loss of dignity, respect, independence and privacy;
- embarrassment relating to bodily functions;
- altered body image;
- strange environments and people;
- worry about catching an infection;
- sensory impairment that might cause communication difficulties;
- attitudes and knowledge of staff;
- denial of basic human needs, such as food, water, warmth and safety.

Clearly, there may be other issues that relate to the experience of anxiety. All of us become anxious at times and it usually due to our perceptions of how well we can cope and whether or not we are in control of a particular situation. Hospitalisation has the potential to generate anxiety because there is a degree of losing control. When one becomes a patient there are certain rules to abide by. Hospitals have their own rules that might, on occasions, be difficult to adhere to. For example, mealtimes will be different and the quality of the food is largely out of one's control. In some instances there are set routines for washing, dressing and going to bed. Although certain elements of individuality can be preserved, hospitals tend to have their own patterns of activity that largely revolve around the admission and discharge of patients.

Hospital wards are in the main busy and impersonal places, for example your bed may be next to that of a complete stranger and at night there is the risk of a lot of noise from people being admitted or telephones ringing and people talking. Therefore, as you can see, the potential for anxiety in the hospital patient is a real problem.

7.6 Recognising and reducing anxiety (page 136)

How would you recognise that someone was anxious? They could be very talkative or unusually quiet. They might be restless and/or sweating. They may lose eye contact easily, might be asking a lot of questions and/or have nervous laughter. They may even complain of being stressed, worried or frightened or in extreme circumstances even threaten to discharge themselves. There are many different signs to watch out for.

How might a nurse help to reduce anxiety in a patient? There are many ways in which this can be done. Being calm, giving information clearly, listening and responding appropriately, being friendly yet professional and respectful, showing compassion and sensitivity in difficult circumstances, and being competent and knowledgeable by answering questions truthfully.

One of the best ways of reducing anxiety in patients is to explain things carefully and provide information on what is going to happen and what needs to be done. This is very important in an emergency situation, where anxieties of both patient and staff will be heightened. If a nurse can empathise with a patient's situation, that is appreciate how it might be affecting them, then it is possible that the nurse will be more effective at reducing anxiety through her or his response (Egan, 1998).

Empathy can be defined as *Seeing another person as oneself, a person* (Northouse, 1979). This definition implies that the person in the bed is just like you or me, one and the same, with an equal propensity for hope, belonging, fear, anxiety, pain and uncertainty at this vulnerable time. Treating a person as you would wish to be treated yourself, if in a similar situation, is generally a good yardstick for the provision of compassionate care.

7.7 'Difficult' patients (page 139)

Again, this is not an easy exercise. Hopefully, you will not hear too many instances of negative labelling during handover. Clearly, there are times when nurses need to be warned of potentially aggressive and dangerous situations because this is of great importance for both staff and patient safety. However, sometimes because of stress and occasional personality clashes, the nurse may inadvertently describe the patient in a negative way that then creates a somewhat false impression of the individual in the minds of others.

It is not possible to like all of the people you meet through nursing and sometimes people in your care may challenge or frustrate you. It is important to be realistic and accept that everyone is different and that illness behaviour can vary from person to person. Some people will be easier to nurse than others because of their attitudes, expectations and coping mechanisms.

In the course of your work as a nurse you must always be alert to this possibility, but never make offensive subjective statements either verbally or in writing about the patients in your care (NMC, 2002a).

7.8 Prejudice and bias (page 139)

You might have recognised the need for:

- self-awareness and recognising one's own prejudices and attitudes towards others;
- fairness and equity – treating people equally;
- listening and responding skills;
- knowledge of cultural and class differences, including religious practices and language;
- open-mindedness;
- empathy and understanding;
- assertiveness;
- challenging other people's attitudes and inappropriate labelling.

Knowledge review

Now that you have read the chapter, how would you rate your knowledge of the following topics?

	Good	Adequate	Poor
1. Expert Patient Programme (EPP)			
2. Patient satisfaction			
3. The 'difficult' patient			
4. Recognising and reducing patient anxiety			

Further reading

Cuthbert, S and Quallington, J (2008) *Values for Care Practice: Health and social care theory and practice.* Exeter: Reflect Press.

Roy, L (2001) *Understanding the Human Rights Act: A toolkit for the health service.* Abingdon: Radcliffe Medical.

Useful websites

www.dh.gov.uk Provides access to the latest policy documents from the Department of Health, including information on the various NSFs, the management of LTCs and the EPP. You will note that there is a continuing theme of patient involvement and participation in the various documents you can access.

www.expertpatients.co.uk Expands upon the DH information on the EPP and provides more detail on how to become an Expert Patient. Clearly outlines the programme's aims and objectives and provides access to the latest news and information. You will find associated links to views from patients and professionals, and there are opportunities for people to join the programme and help others with their management of LTCs.

www.ltca.org.uk Interesting website providing information and advice for people with LTCs. The Long Term Conditions Alliance is a UK charity and is the umbrella body for voluntary organisations in the UK that are working to meet the needs of people with LTCs.

www.nmc-uk.org Website of the governing professional body for nurses and midwives, providing up-to-date information on the latest professional developments. You can access and download documents, such as the 2008 *Code of Professional Conduct*, and advice on professional matters. The various publications of the NMC on professional issues, such as confidentiality and record keeping, can be accessed.

www.patients-association.org.uk Interesting website for healthcare users. Contains up-to-date information about patients' rights and gives opportunities for people to raise concerns and share experiences. The Patients' Association is a national charity that produces reports, and offers help and advice. The site provides access to weekly news reports and there is an online forum for patients to discuss problems and explore possible solutions.

Chapter 8

The student experience

NMC Standards of Proficiency

This chapter will address the following NMC *Standards of Proficiency* and *Outcomes to be achieved for entry to the branch programme*.

Manage oneself, one's practice, and that of others, in accordance with *The NMC Code of Professional Conduct: Standards for conduct, performance and ethics*, recognising one's own abilities and limitations.

Outcomes to be achieved for entry to the branch programme:
Discuss in an informed manner the implications of professional regulation for nursing practice:

- demonstrate a basic knowledge of professional regulation and self-regulation;
- recognise and acknowledge the limitations of one's own abilities;
- recognise situations that require referral to a registered practitioner.

Demonstrate an awareness of the NMC Code of Professional Conduct: Standards for conduct, performance and ethics:

- commit to the principle that the primary purpose of the registered nurse is to protect and serve society;
- accept responsibility for one's own actions and decisions.

Demonstrate a commitment to the need for continuing professional development and personal supervision activities in order to enhance knowledge, skills, values and attitudes needed for safe and effective nursing practice.

Outcomes to be achieved for entry to the branch programme:
Demonstrate responsibility for one's own learning through the development of a portfolio of practice and recognise when further learning is required:

- identify specific learning needs and objectives;
- begin to engage with, and interpret, the evidence base which underpins nursing practice.

Acknowledge the importance of seeking supervision to develop safe and effective nursing practice.

Chapter aims

After reading this chapter, you will able to:

- understand how to become an active learner by utilising a range of study skills;
- understand the implications of professional regulation for registered practitioners;
- discuss how your learning in practice (in order to meet the NMC standards of proficiency) can be achieved;
- consider how you can manage challenges in your work/life balance when undertaking your course.

Introduction

This chapter explores the student experience and considers what it means to be a nursing student in a university. Healthcare and, in particular, nursing students will have a different experience from other university students, partly because of the compulsory clinical practice element and partly because of the responsibilities associated with the levels of accountability and responsibility of becoming a professional nurse. This has implications for working in practice areas with other professionals, service users and their carers and families, and this chapter will spend some time focusing on these issues for you as a student.

The experience of being in a university is also an exciting and challenging experience for students, from starting nursing programmes and meeting new colleagues to managing their learning experiences over the three years of a programme. This chapter will explore in more detail the study skills required to achieve this: undertaking assessments in practice, working with mentors and how to achieve the competences necessary for registration with the NMC.

Starting university

The move into universities for nursing has several benefits for the development of nursing as a profession and reflects the future changing workforce needs of the NHS. In many universities nursing is now taught alongside other professions allied to medicine (such as physiotherapy, occupational therapy or dietetics) in an inter-professional and interdisciplinary way that mirrors the way in which care is delivered in practice. It is important that nurses, as professionals, explore the specific nursing knowledge and the values that underpin nursing care in practice in whatever pathway they have chosen. This does not mean that we should ever lose sight of the overall aim of all health professionals, which is to care for the individual's health needs.

Knowledge for nursing practice is developed through a variety of sources, from evidence gained through research and scholarship, to practical knowledge, to individuals' knowledge acquired through their own personal and professional experience (Cronin and Rawlings-Anderson, 2004). The aim is to develop competent and confident registered practitioners who are both 'fit for practice' and 'fit for purpose', and are able to function in a variety of care settings that will evolve through the twenty-first century. The NMC has also considered fitness for the award that you will have achieved at the end of your course. You will then be able to demonstrate how you have developed the necessary knowledge and practice to enable you to become a registered nurse (NMC, 2002b).

Coming to study at university can initially be a very daunting experience for new students; nursing students enter education through a wide variety of routes, such as access to HE courses as well as A levels or their equivalent. Students come from many different backgrounds and have different life experiences. This enables those coming into nursing to both reflect the population they will care for and offer a breadth of experience, skills and knowledge that can only enhance their learning and contribute to the academic community they have joined.

However, if your experience of school was less positive than others in your group, or career or family commitments have prevented you from starting a nursing course earlier in your life, you may lack confidence and feel anxious about the whole experience. You have, however, successfully jumped the first hurdle on the road to becoming a registered nurse by being accepted onto your chosen course: this is recognition of the potential you already have. You will experience the huge social change in those who opt to go to university as part of their professional education and the ongoing change this will bring to employment opportunities and potential and lifestyle (HEFC, 2001).

Activity 8.1

It can be useful to think through the hopes and fears you may have about studying at university (we shall consider practice experience later on), and these may range from meeting new people, to moving away from home, to how to write an assignment.

With a friend or colleague from your group, take five minutes to write down:

- **what hopes and fears you have about studying at university;**
- **what resources both socially and personally you already have in place.**

Discuss these lists with your friend or colleague.

Keep these two lists and look at them again at the end of the chapter. It often helps to be able to write down specific points such as 'fear of the unknown' as, instead of feeling alone and overwhelmed by the experience, you can see that you are not, because others in your group may have exactly the same fears as you. Writing them down often makes them appear less frightening, and some of the fears may have an easy solution after discussion, either with your group and with your tutor.

As this activity is based on your own feelings, there is no outline answer at the end of the chapter.

Universities have many resources in place to help new students and also many other opportunities available that will enhance your whole experience, and be a source of support to you in the more challenging times during the three years on the course, such as the anxiety of starting in new teams on practice, or submitting your academic work for the first time. One resource, for example, is freshers' week, where some new students can meet and be introduced to the social and cultural life that the university offers. Activities are provided all week by the different university societies, sports clubs, the students union and other university services such as the chaplaincy. These will introduce you to the opportunities available for you to participate in student life as well as make new friends and learn new skills. Many universities offer a 'buddy' system, where second- and third-year students mentor first-year students during the first few weeks, offering the support you may need during this new and exciting time. Some students may feel like 'fish out of water' during their first few weeks on the course, so give yourself time to settle down, meet and make new friends, and adjust to the changes that your family and friends will see in you during your course.

In the first few weeks you will be given a personal tutor. This role can vary from university to university; however, the common factor is the consistency of support that the tutor can offer you throughout your programme. There are many different roles that the personal tutor can undertake. They will see you regularly throughout your course and be there as a source of support, academic advice and professional development, and as an advocate who will work with you to achieve your outcomes for the course. The main role of the personal tutor is to make sure that you have completed all your academic work successfully, have achieved the competences for registration, and have met the requirements of the NMC. He or she is an important person for you to work with and seek support from; the personal tutor sees you as an individual and offers pastoral as well as academic guidance, and should be your first port of call when you feel you need help. The relationship that you may have with them as an adult is different from the teacher–pupil relationship that you may have recently (or not so recently) experienced at school. Tutors aim to work with their personal students, be challenged by them and guide them throughout the three years towards registration. They are there to nurture you and are able to offer strategies to help you learn and develop as a professional nurse. In the first few weeks of the course it is important that you meet together to begin this relationship; this means that the tutor can start to get to know you as a person and any specific needs you may have, so that they can help and direct you in meeting these.

Becoming a nursing student

All nursing students undertake their education in universities where 50 per cent of their time is spent on theoretical aspects of their course and 50 per cent in clinical practice. Clinical practice placements are undertaken in the local Acute Care Trusts, Primary Care Trusts and the independent sectors. These are the private healthcare facilities, charitable trusts and others, such as hospices, who provide care for a wide range of clients and their families. All these placements provide a wealth of learning opportunities for students, who can develop a wide range of skills enabling them to work with a range of different client groups. There are two routes to obtaining registration: a diploma in HE or a degree in nursing, with eligibility to register with the NMC. Both these routes take three years and the same number of practice and theory hours are required by the NMC. This is currently 2,300 hours in theory and 2,300 hours in practice over three years; however, 300 hours in practice may be achieved through clinical skills simulation and practice in clinical skills laboratories (NMC, 2006a).

Three-year programmes consist of one year of a Common Foundation Programme (CFP), and two years of the chosen branch. Each student is required to successfully pass the CFP before they are able to progress to their branch programme. This is something you need to be aware of as the NMC does not allow students to continue their education into the branch programme unless all outcomes for the CFP have been achieved and confirmed within twelve weeks of entering the branch programme (NMC, 2006b). Thus, you may have to withdraw and rejoin another cohort until this requirement has been met. The CFP allows students to have a taste of what nursing in other branches entails during this year – for example, you may undertake some theory and practice in mental health nursing even though you have chosen to become an adult nurse. The aim is for all students to have an appreciation of the needs of clients, service users and their families throughout the whole life span.

Adult nurses are required to meet in theory and practice European directives (EU) 77/453/EEC and 89/595/EEC. These are a mandatory part of all adult nursing programmes. The NMC ensures that all approved programmes for the education of nurses meet these requirements in the number of hours in theory and practice they are required to undertake, and the content and practice experience they will require in meeting these. Universities offer a variety of ways in which they ensure that these requirements are met from undertaking practical experience – for example, in mental health nursing and maternity care to working with other health professionals under the appropriate supervisors of practice (NMC, 2006b).

The CFP has theoretical and clinical skills-based objectives to achieve and asks the student to demonstrate by the end of the year the theoretical and practical knowledge that contributes to the care and well-being of clients in such subjects as psychology and sociology, as well as health promotion and education, and physiology. Fundamental nursing care and practical skills acquisition form a key part of this year, with students learning, for example, how to administer medication safely and how to calculate drug dosages. Integral to the acquisition of these skills are the essential skills clusters (ESCs) – a set of clinical skills that are essential for both the CFP and branch programmes. They have been introduced explicitly into nursing programmes as a result of public concern about the safety of patients (NMC, 2007a). The ESC consider important aspects of skill acquisition such as care, compassion and communication, organisational aspects of care, infection prevention and control, nutrition and fluid management, and medicines management. These are all skills you will undertake during your first year and subsequent branch programme. It is important to remember that professional nursing is a three-year programme and you will be expected to work towards achieving the proficiencies required for registration: this is a gradual process and you will have achieved this by the end of three years. Remember that the patient, client or service user is the person who is central to the care you give and their health, welfare and safety are paramount.

Profession or occupation?

Nursing is a legally regulated profession through the NMC, established by Act of Parliament in 2002. This entitles registered practitioners to use the title Registered Nurse, Midwife or Specialist Community Public Health Nurse. As a professional the nurse is therefore accountable to the public, to the professional body (the NMC), to their patients and to their employer. The NMC is not purely for the registration of nursing and midwifery practitioners, but has several other functions related to setting standards for the practice and education of its registrants and would-be registrants. These standards are the core principles by which nursing practice is judged and the *NMC Code of Professional Conduct* (2008) enables practitioners to be able to state explicitly the boundaries of nursing practice. The *Code* has recently been reviewed to include the words 'performance' and 'ethics', thereby making it clear what the public can expect from a professional nurse. These are such key principles as respect, consent, confidentiality and the maintenance of competence and knowledge for practice.

This makes the assumption that nursing is a profession and has the characteristics of a profession; these characteristics are what gives nursing its authority to practice in a way that fulfils its obligations to society and to the patients, users, carers and families.

Sociologists have defined professions and their role in society, and have considered what constitutes a profession. There is a general agreement among sociologists about what the key characteristics of a profession are. Eraut (1994) has discussed the emergence in particular of those professions that are closely allied to medicine, including nursing, and has identified the following characteristics of professions.

- A unique body of knowledge: this is closely aligned with how this knowledge is transmitted to those who wish to enter the profession. This can be through a period of internship in which the student spends a significant amount of time learning their 'craft' and is under the close supervision of an expert practitioner. It is always in an HE context and there are significant hoops to jump through on the journey to registration and the exclusivity that this provides.
- A strong service ideal, whereby the well-being of the client is of primary importance.
- Professions are able to exercise autonomy and control in their care of clients and have developed ethical codes and frameworks to be able to justify decisions and exercise accountability in doing so.

If we consider the above characteristics of a profession we can see that nursing goes part of the way towards meeting some of these criteria, but is prevented from doing so because nursing is still evolving a substantive body of nursing knowledge. Although, as we have identified, nurse education is now firmly embedded in universities, the majority of nurses qualify at diploma rather than at graduate level, which suggests that not all nurses aspire to a true professional status. The NMC is currently undertaking a review of pre-registration curricula in which one proposal is for an all-graduate profession; if adopted, this will have a considerable impact both on entrants to nursing and on workforce development: the question is, will this lead to an elite nursing profession and, if so, will this be a good thing for patient care?

Where does nursing knowledge come from?

There have been many theorists in nursing over the past 30 years who have considered the nature of the knowledge that supports nursing practice (Benner, 1984; Carper, 1978).

Richardson et al. (2004), however, take a more pragmatic view about practice knowledge, which incorporates not just nursing but all practitioners and clients involved in patients' care. The authors articulate the dynamic nature of knowledge in response to the changing social and cultural needs of patients and clients. Gustavsson (2004) identifies three forms of knowledge:

- **Epistome**. This is about the scientific form of knowledge and is based on proof and fact. Think about EBP (see Chapter 5) and you will see that this is the type of knowledge that Gustavsson is talking about. Epistome is highly valued among some members of the health community.
- **Techne**. This is about practical knowledge – what we actually do as nurses. It is more complex in that it explores our ability to solve problems when confronted by new experiences. It looks at knowing how we do things and why we do things. An experienced nurse, for example, will not only know *how* to take a temperature but *why*, and will know the consequences for the patient if this is found to be abnormal. Techne allows the practitioner to apply theory to practice situations, which in nursing is important if you are to develop into a qualified practitioner, as it will not be enough to know just how to do things, but also why you do them.
- **Phronesis**. Also known as tacit knowledge, this is the knowledge that we bring to a situation from our own experience as a nurse and as a person. This also implies that what we do has an ethical component, as we are aware of the results of our actions and their effects upon others.

Activity 8.2

Think of a patient or client you have nursed: what sort of knowledge did you or your mentor use to care for this patient?

A brief outline answer is provided at the end of the chapter.

How skill and competence can be developed in nursing

Once you have considered what sort of knowledge begins to explain and underpin nursing practice, it is useful to think about how clinical competence can be acquired and judged. Nursing is a practice-based profession and the skills development in whatever branch you follow will always be an important part of the assessment process.

Benner (1984) developed a linear theory to explain how nurses develop practical skills and move from being novice practitioners to becoming expert practitioners.

- **Novices** have no practical experience of the situation in which they will perform. Novices need rules and guidelines as their inexperience means that they are limited in their ability to make sense of some situations.
- **Advanced beginners** are those nurses who are experienced enough in real situations to be able to recognise recurring patterns in a clinical situation, but who still require rules and guidelines to inform their practice.
- **Competent practitioners** are those who have had two to three years' experience and who can plan methodically and logically in given situations. They recognise patterns of illness and behaviour in patients, for example a patient who is depressed.
- **Proficient practitioners** are those who are able to assimilate situations and see the whole picture, rather than the snapshot of the competent practitioner. At this level nurses have developed good decision-making skills.
- **Expert nurses** are able to focus on the problem presented and are able to use tacit knowledge to sort the 'wheat from the chaff' in dealing with patients' conditions and problems.

Activity 8.3

Think about your own experience and assess where you are according to Benner. Discuss this with someone in your class.

- How did you decide where to categorise yourself, and why did you choose that level?
- Can you think of an example in your life where you are now an expert but were a novice, and how you progressed through to your current level of expertise?

Benner's work is important as it helps to clarify for students that the development of professional skills and competence is an ongoing and continuous development throughout their working lives.

As this activity is based on your own experience, there is no outline answer at the end of the chapter.

Being professional

The professional status accorded to registered nurses carries with it some prerequisites for the behaviour and roles of a professional nurse, so that nurses can be accountable for their actions and decisions. In order for the nurse to exercise this accountability there are several associated aspects: responsibility, competence, authority and autonomy (Cronin and Rawlings-Anderson, 2004).

- **Responsibility** is undertaken and accepted by nurses as part of their everyday practice, and may be for others within that sphere, such as student nurses.

Nurses are responsible for the interventions that fall into the domain of nursing practice and need to be aware of those duties that fall outside a nurse's level of competence.

- **Competence** has been discussed previously in relation to Benner; however, it is worth noting that student nurses are expected to be competent and fit for purpose at the point of registration and it is the duty of all registered nurses to maintain their professional knowledge and competence in order to register annually to practice.
- **Authority** is vested in nurses in a variety of ways through knowledge, skills and position; for example, a Matron who has responsibility for and authority over a clinical area.
- **Autonomy** is problematic in nursing: if a nurse is responsible enough to carry out care and has both the competence and authority to do this, individual practitioners' autonomy should naturally follow on. This will enable the nurse to accept both responsibility and accountability for their actions. Nurses are hampered by regulation and through other professions such as medicine, which limit nurses' autonomy to practise effectively. This aspect of professional practice is, however, being addressed by the new roles taken on by nurses and the associated responsibility that this carries, for example the role of Nurse Consultant (see Chapters 2 and 3).

The above discussion should indicate the complexity of nursing practice in modern healthcare for all practitioners and students.

How does this apply to me as a student?

At the beginning of this section it was identified that the NMC sets standards for practice and how these can be incorporated into practice. As befits a profession, these standards are reviewed regularly to incorporate any changes in legislation, for example the Mental Capacity Act (2005), or changes in non-medical prescribing. The onus is on the nurse to both maintain these standards and abide by the *Code of Professional Conduct*; the responsibility and accountability for their own practice is a key task for all registered practitioners and one that all nursing students should be aware of.

The concept of knowing your own boundaries and limitations is important on your journey towards becoming a registered practitioner. This may relate to care you haven't delivered before, types of medical conditions you have not met, a lack of knowledge about a particular issue or uncertainty as to how to calculate a drug dosage for a child. All these areas can put a patient at risk, and it is important that you are aware of your own limitations when in practice. Your colleagues and mentors are aware that you may be unsure of what are your limitations, but they are there to help you put into context the parameters you will work within and it is important that these are discussed when you are in practice, so that you feel confident in delivering care safely and competently. When in doubt always speak to the registered practitioner who will be able to advise, support and help you in learning to be able to manage care competently, confidently and safely.

Activity 8.4

Although you may have had limited contact with your chosen client groups, it is useful to consider the implications for professional practice and registration of the *Code of Professional Conduct* (NMC, 2008). In pairs with another student nurse (not necessarily in your chosen pathway):

* find out what part of the register you will both be on when you qualify and describe how you did this;
* read the Code of Professional Conduct's standards for conduct, performance and ethics;
* consider the standards that discuss accountability for your individual practice and for ensuring that anti-discriminatory practice is delivered; then think of a client you have each cared for individually and discuss how these two standards were demonstrated in the care given to those clients.

There is a brief outline answer at the end of the chapter.

Developing lifelong study skills

Developing good study skills and habits will enable you to:

* be successful;
* be less stressed;
* plan your time effectively so that you can enjoy your life;
* plan for all types of assessment;
* achieve your goal of becoming a registered nurse.

Study skills, like any others, can be learnt and practised and, if worked on steadily, can make you a happier and more successful student. Effective and successful students are made not born, according to Burns and Sinfield (2003). It is important to remember this and not to dwell on your past experience of education, if this has not been an enjoyable or fruitful experience. Remember, nursing is a combination of practical skills and the application of theory and it is theory that supports your practice. Nurses currently in practice have continuously to maintain their knowledge and skills in order to re-register annually with the NMC, so by becoming an effective and efficient learner you are going to equip yourself with a lifelong skill that will be integral to your future career and employment.

Your university will have a learning and development department as part of their learning resources and this will be a source of excellent tips, help and support to all students during their time at university, so don't be shy of seeking help from them at any point in your course. For some students going to university may reveal a special learning need, such as dyslexia. There are tutors whose expertise is in learning and development and who will be able to help you and give you support in cases such as this. In some cases financial help is available for the purchase of equipment to aid you in your course work.

Becoming an active learner

One of the outcomes for this chapter is to become an active learner: this is a learner who actively seeks out ways to develop their own knowledge; who tries to make sense of complex concepts by undertaking learning activities that enhance their knowledge; and who seeks out deeper rather than surface learning. Such learners are characterised by being enthusiastic about their chosen subject; reflecting on their work and actions; having a level of self-awareness and constantly evaluating themselves against the goals they are trying to achieve; generally having a good attention span; and having the ability to apply learning to various situations. You will note that this is not a picture of a passive person who doesn't engage with learning, doesn't reflect and may become easily bored. This is as important for academic skills as it is for undertaking learning in the practice area.

Research by Burns and Sinfield (2003) demonstrates that active learners have a much higher level of learning and thus develop the ability to move on from merely repeating information in a set format, as, for example, you may do for an exam in your first year, to being able to apply a theory to a number of complex situations. The development of this skill is essential if you are to be successful as a registered nurse, and able to deal with the many complex and challenging situations you will face on a daily basis. For example, you may learn the theory of respiration and the structure and function of the lungs in what is termed surface learning, but active learners will go on to develop how to apply this theory to a range of patients, for example a child with asthma or an adult with bronchitis.

Finding out your preferred learning style

The first step is to consider what type of learning style suits you and what is your preferred way of learning, as there are many. Cottrell (1999) gives an overview of learning styles questionnaires, for example Honey and Mumford (2006), Kolb (1984) and the VARK (visual, aural, read/write and kinesthetic) (www.vark-learn.com). To identify your own individual learning style, a quick and easy approach is to consider the concept of 'see, hear and do' in relation to learning: this considers which of the three styles a learner relies upon predominantly when engaged in learning.

- **See**: this is for people who learn best by using a visual approach, for example by watching a demonstration of a skill.
- **Hear**: this is for people who learn best by hearing, for example an explanation of how the heart works.
- **Do**: this is for people who learn best by doing, for example giving an injection.

It is important that you identify which type of learning style is your preferred way to learn, as by doing this you can consider techniques to become an active and more effective learner. By identifying your preferred style you will find the material you are going to explore will be more relevant, interesting and easier to learn .

Activity 8.5

Find some of the learning style questionnaires on the internet, which are fun to complete as well as being of practical help to you.

* Go to www.agelesslearner.com or www.bbc.co.uk/keyskills and complete their learning styles questionnaires. Some may find that they have a strong preference for one particular style, but most people use a variety of styles to adapt to different situations.

As this is a practical activity, there is no outline answer at the end of the chapter.

Garrett and Clarke (2008) suggest some techniques to use once you have discovered your preferred learning style.

* **Visual learners**. Sit at the front of the class, so that the teacher's expressions, facial cues and body language can be seen. Make detailed notes in class, and use pictures, drawings and diagrams to help you make sense of more complex concepts. Use visualisation to help you think about more abstract concepts, for example depression.
* **Auditory learners**. Sit where you can clearly hear the teacher, or your group if this is a seminar presentation, as speech, vocal pitch and tone help you to assimilate material. Record lectures or use the podcasts provided to listen. Detailed note taking is not the most effective way for you to learn and this may be of limited use to you in some situations, for example lectures. Work in groups so that you can discuss material with colleagues and teachers.
* **Tactile learners**. The trick for you is to avoid boredom from sitting too long without something practical to occupy you during lectures. Use a highlighter when you make notes in class and transfer these later to notebooks or your PC. Draw relevant and appropriate pictures when studying, such as a diagram of the heart.

Environment

Much of the work you will undertake at university will be done alongside other students in classrooms and lecture theatres; however, you will also need to work independently on activities such as reading, revision for exams and writing assignments. The place where you do this needs to be comfortable, warm and free from distraction, and it should have some space where you can spread out your books, papers and anything else that you feel helps you when completing your work; also make sure you have a comfortable chair to sit on. It may be the place where you have your personal computer; it can be your bedroom or a designated study space in your house. This sets the tempo and scene for studying, writing and reflection. If you try to study where there are constant distractions, such as noise, television and where even the ironing can appear more attractive on the occasions when you do not feel motivated to study, these distractions can become what are known as displacement activities and will prevent you achieving your goals, as you will not establish an effective study routine.

It is worth thinking about where and when you are going to study effectively as soon as you have been accepted for a place on your chosen course. Some students find the university library a good venue: it is quiet and warm, and has space and desks for you to work on. It puts you in a 'work mode' and three hours spent in a library can often be more productive than a day at home. Establish a set of ground rules for your family or housemates when you want to study, for example no interruptions for an hour, or no loud music for three hours. Some students have found different times of the day more conducive to study than others, for example early morning before everyone else in your house has risen for the day. It is important that your study time is protected as this is the key to your success and it helps to share with your partners, family and housemates the reason why this is important to you in reaching your goals.

All students will be expected to have acquired basic computer literacy skills by the end of the CFP programme. This will include being able to send and receive emails, submit a word-processed assignment, and use the university intranet. This will be a steep learning curve for some, but it will be essential if you are to be able to be successful in participating fully in electronic forms of learning such as webcasting, podcasting, online discussion groups, wikis and blogs. Your university will have as part of its learning and development team tutors who will be able to help you with getting to grips with these new skills.

Time management

It is worth stating the obvious to say that study takes time: for each hour's lecture you go to, you need to do about three hours of effective study alongside this. This translates into about nine hours of independent study time on top of the hours you are required to attend university. It is easy to say 'I don't have time to learn study skills', but these will save you time in the long run by making you a more effective and efficient learner. Some students already have good time management skills and have previously managed to juggle home, family and a job. When you start your course review this situation and reflect on your own skills of time management. This is an area where you as a student already have some transferable skills, whether it was to get to work on time or in organising your own life. Starting a course such as nursing can make you feel like a complete novice, and in many aspects of care you will be; however, this is one area where most people have already got some skills, so be positive!

Activity 8.6

You need to undertake this activity in a group of five people. A week consists of 168 hours and it is worth writing down how you spend yours.

- As an individual write down the number of hours you spend each week on: personal hygiene, eating, cooking, shopping, working, hobbies, routine chores, playing, socialising, travelling and, of course, sleeping.

Activity 8.6 continued

- As a group, discuss what time management problems you can foresee, such as dealing with a sick child. Write these down and as a group offer practical solutions about how you would deal with these.
- How many hours does all this add up to and what time is left for study? Discuss with your group the issues that arose and what solutions people can offer for those who appear to have very little time for study in their packed week.

As this is a practical activity, there is no outline answer at the end of the chapter.

Already you have an awareness that you do need to plan your time to be successful and to ensure that you meet the goals and deadlines set for your assignments. There are various techniques you can use to make sure you use your time productively and effectively.

- **Little and often**. Develop a routine, studying at the same time each day and for a set period; it then does not become a chore but is incorporated into your lifestyle and you maintain your motivation to study.
- **Rewards**. Give yourself a regular break for a drink or something to eat; most people cannot concentrate on one thing for longer than 20 minutes continuously, and thus it is important that your study routine involves a variety of study techniques from reading to note taking to watching a film, in order to maintain your concentration, keep you motivated and help you to retain information and learn more effectively.
- **Consider temperament and learning style**. Is there an optimum time of day for you to study, when your energy and concentration are high; for example, are you a morning person? You can then plan to do the most challenging parts of studying at this time. If you attempt this when you are not at your best and your energy levels are low, you will quickly become demotivated and disheartened.
- **Keep a diary**. Many shops sell academic diaries that run from August until July as well as yearly wall planners. These serve as visual reminders of the tasks for the year and the course assignment deadlines you have to meet, plus things like holidays, term times and family commitments such as weddings. Putting these in allows you to plan your work and study schedule so that you are able to achieve the outcomes for the year at a steady pace; this will undoubtedly cause you less stress in the long run and will increase your chances of success.
- **Avoid cramming and 'going down to the wire'**. These are the least successful methods of achieving success and are to be avoided. Cramming for exams does not allow you to retain information in a logical way; instead, when you go in to take a exam, it increases the risk of failure as you have not learnt and assimilated the material. 'Going down to the wire' and completing work an hour before handing it in means that you are not alert enough to think logically and coherently – again, a recipe for failure. These two strategies are counter-productive and in the long run will cause you stress and increase your chances of failure. You have been warned!

Reading effectively

It would be impossible to read all the textbooks, journals, newspapers and internet pages recommended to you during your course, as well as undertake the reading required to complete your assignments. In general, students spend too much time reading texts that are not relevant to their assignments or the work they are undertaking. Reading at HE level means that you have to read some essential texts and research in detail, while other texts that are useful to you will have to be read selectively. This does not mean that you can get by reading as little as possible, as you will never become an active learner and be able to demonstrate a depth as well as a breadth of knowledge when writing your assignments or engaging in practice. The skill is in recognising the different forms that reading takes and adapting your study time effectively to enable you to do this.

Why am I reading?

Think about the purpose of your reading; is it:

- to find information or consider a specific fact, such as the side effects of a particular drug;
- to find out how to undertake a skill;
- for revision;
- for an assignment that requires the current available evidence to support your work;
- to find out about current government policies or relevant health or social care?

Selecting the texts you want takes time, as you need to search databases and look in the library at each book before you decide what is relevant or not to your chosen topic. You will need to factor this in when you start your assignments or when you are reading to support your work, for example participation in a group seminar. Get to know your library and the subject librarian for health as they are an invaluable source of information about the latest texts tutors recommend for their particular subjects. Reading an academic text for the first time may be frightening and anxiety-provoking, particularly if you don't feel that you understand anything the first time you read through it. Practice does, however, make perfect and by following the tips below you will find that you will increase in confidence and competence in reading for your course.

Sifting 'the wheat from the chaff'

The first stage for developing reading skills is to select the texts you are going to read. You can do this from reading lists given to you by your tutors or through searching the library catalogues or the many online databases available, such as CINHAL or Medline. It is then important to gain an overview of how useful the book is for you: for example, does it contain the right information, is it at the right level, is it up to date? This last point is particularly important in nursing practice as the information in books more than five years old may have been superseded by developments in medicine and healthcare.

Look at how the book is structured:

- the author's name and whether he or she is well known in the field;
- the title page and the list of contents;
- any opening introductory chapters explaining the contents.

By a brief consideration of the above you can quickly begin to see if the book will be useful for you, but by not spending time doing this you run the risk of ordering books from your library that may have promising titles but bear no relation to the subject you are interested in.

The same principle applies to journal articles: once you have undertaken a literature search and have a selection of articles, before you order any or print any off look at the abstract, read the first and last paragraphs and evaluate if you think the article is relevant for you.

Nursing and healthcare textbooks need to be read in a different way to be able to learn and make sense of them. Being an active learner using the SQ3R strategy developed by Rowntree (1998) enables you engage with reading in a meaningful way. Before you start your reading have a list of questions in your head about what you want from the text.

- **S** is for Surveying: this is the technique identified at the beginning of this paragraph – skim read the text and the first and last paragraphs.
- **Q** is for Questions: an active learner attempts to read critically and asks questions while reading; this may be as basic as 'How?' or 'Why?', but as you start to read in more depth these may change to more focused questions, such as 'What is the evidence for this assumption?'
- **R** is for Read: take time to read more slowly and at a more even pace to take in the information, especially more complex texts. Adopt the 'washing an elephant' approach – a bit at a time; this may be a paragraph or a page. This requires concentration and putting into practice the preparation of the environment and time management skills discussed previously.
- **R** is for Recite/Recall: after reading put aside the text and try to recall what was said, the meaning and any questions that arose while you were reading; finally, ask yourself if you can make use of it. For most students it is helpful to make notes so that you can later go back and review these for the purpose of assignment writing or examinations and to clarify in your own mind what you have learnt.
- **R** is for Review: go back and look at the piece you have read. Are all your questions answered, and do you understand the concepts and information?

These five steps can seem quite laborious when you first attempt a more active approach to reading, but, like all skills, you will improve with practice and will be able to read more quickly and, more importantly, more effectively by the end of the CFP. Of all the study skills, reading effectively is the one that will help you now and in all your future work. As you progress through the course, the ability to read effectively saves you time, enables you to assimilate more complex ideas and, as the level of your academic work increases, enables you to read confidently difficult texts and journals.

Assessments

Assessment is probably the least favourite part of the course, but is necessary in order for you to demonstrate knowledge and understanding for safe, effective and competent practice. Throughout your course you will be assessed in both theory and practice.

Courses will have a range of types of assignments, usually including essays, examinations, multiple-choice questions, presentations, poster presentations, objective structured clinical examinations (OSCEs) and, for those undertaking degree studies, a project or a research proposal.

The main areas for assessment are the essay and, to a lesser extent, exams. In looking at more detail about planning your work, you can see that much of the success in this can be learnt through applying a basic set of principles to writing your assignment that will increase your success and marks. As with all aspects of learning in this chapter this involves you becoming an active learner.

Essays and other written work

There are three main types of written work you will be asked to produce (Magne, 2004).

- **The reflection.** This is about your own experience and development, and often forms part of an essay or is useful for your portfolio work. It is usually written in the first person, demonstrates your own thoughts and feelings, and is often personal in nature. This is useful for you as a student in developing self-awareness and a deeper insight of the care you have given to a patient or client. There are many forms of reflective cycles; however, Gibbs (1998) is the most commonly used and offers several ways in which this can be developed as a form of learning.
- **Research reviews and comparisons.** All of you will at some point be asked to review, critique, contrast or compare pieces of research and there is a formal structure that allows you to do this; for example, Parahoo (2006) and Cormack (2006) will both be able to offer frameworks for this. Reviews and comparisons are formal pieces of work using the third person and demonstrate different levels of knowledge throughout your course. This is an essential skill to master, both for your course and for your future career, where you may be asked to do something similar when comparing approaches to care or considering implementing new innovations in practice.
- **The research-based assignment.** This is an essay that is related to the module that you are undertaking. It is expected that students will have to search and read the current research and texts on the chosen topic, and it involves you being able to read, understand and offer different views and comparisons. Crucially, to complete these successfully you must have looked at a range of people's works and opinions, from government reports to original pieces of research. This is the most common type of essay you will be asked for, but is challenging to write and can at first seem quite daunting.

Review the previous paragraphs on reading and preparation. You will be given your essay title in the first few days of the module as well as a schedule for when tutorials are arranged, so put these in your diary. Make an appointment to see the lecturer, and then work out a timetable for you to complete the work by, making sure this is at least five days before the due date.

The essay question

Analysis of the essay question, which can be done in groups or with a friend, helps you to be clear about the subject, the parameters of this and what you know already about this area. It will also direct you to the type of research you need to look at and the books that may be helpful. When we talked about active reading we looked at targeting your reading and having a list of questions for when you read. You can see that, if you do this preliminary stage, you are already saving time and becoming an active learner.

Activity 8.7

Here is the title of an essay that could be given to CFP students:

Communication is the most important aspect of caring for patients; discuss this statement.

In a pair with a member from your group discuss this title and start to plan how you would write the essay. Make a list of aspects that you would need to consider.

There is a brief outline answer at the end of the chapter.

Planning the writing

The hard work comes next when you need to actually do the searching and the reading; however, this is the foundation on which your essay will be built.

Essays consist of three main parts.

- **The introduction**. This is best written last as you can then check the key points of the essay. Students often neglect the introduction and merely repeat the question; however, a good introduction grabs your reader straightaway so that they want to read on – they want to hear your arguments and to know what you think.

  Tell them what you are going to tell them, and use short sentences to point them in the right direction – this is known as signposting and really offers a list of headings for the reader so that they know what you are going to discuss and in what order. Summarise the content and, if the set question asks you to do so, offer rationales for why you have adopted this approach. Set the parameters of your arguments; for example, if your essay is about communication, you might confine this to verbal communication as opposed to written or non-verbal communication.

- **The main body**. This is the part of the essay that presents your arguments, so present them in a logical way that enables the reader to follow them. Each paragraph should address a new point or topic and, if you are presenting something quite complex, you may need several paragraphs for this. It is important that you understand what you have written and the terminology and concepts you have used. It is very easy to get carried away and try to impress the reader by using complex language that you do not understand – this becomes apparent when your tutor marks the work, and he or she will know that you don't understand the issues under discussion.
- **Conclusion**. The conclusion is equally as important as the introduction and just as neglected by students. Tell them what you've just discussed – the conclusion should summarise your arguments and offer some thoughts about your topic from your reading and writing of the assignment. It should neatly finish off your work. Students make mistakes by not actually concluding the essay, or introducing the key material into the conclusion in one sentence, or introducing a paragraph of new material into the conclusion. These mistakes are costly as they may mean that you do not answer the question or have missed the opportunity to discuss some key issues in your essay.

Final steps

- Write a detailed plan with headings for each paragraph. Show this to your tutor; most universities have a policy stipulating that tutors do not read drafts of undergraduate work, but will read essay plans and samples of work of about a page of A4 in length. A good detailed plan will demonstrate to your tutor your thoughts, ideas and arguments, and is much more helpful than a sample of a page from your essay. Sometimes the plan may be interesting, but the rest of the work does not match up to that, and the student may fail the assignment even though they have shown the plan to the tutor.
- Write your first draft. This takes different people varying amounts of time – you are the only one who knows how quickly you write, so plan your work.
- Put the assignment away and out of sight for about a day. Put some distance between you and your work, as this space gives you time to go back and see factual mistakes and spelling and grammatical errors, and to change the order of your work if this helps the work to flow better. If possible, get someone to read it through for you – they don't have to be a nurse; your parents, partner or a friend will do, as they can tell you if it makes sense or reads correctly.
- Finalise your essay, leaving the introduction until last.
- Put it away again for about a day and take time to reflect on your work. Is it as good as you can make it? Does it say what you want it to say? Does it answer the set question? Does it meet the word limit? Have you referenced it correctly?
- Submit your work.
- Review the feedback you receive. Feedback is crucial if you are to improve your work. Note what the lecturer has said and, if there are comments you don't understand, make an appointment to see him or her. Feedback should praise the work you have done, give you indicators for improvement and give you confidence that all the hard work you have put in has paid off in the mark you receive (Magne, 2004).

Referencing

Referencing is an important aspect of your work, as references demonstrate that you have read about and around the topic and also support the arguments you have made. It is important to reference correctly and your university will have guidelines on their preferred style. The currency of the references is also important and using literature that is contemporary enhances both the accuracy and content of your work.

Exams

Examinations are there to test your knowledge and, later on, if you have exams in the second and third years, they demonstrate application and some critical reflection and are not just a showcase for what you know.

Preparation

Preparation is just as important for exams as it is for essay writing; we have looked at cramming as not being a helpful or, in the long run, successful way to pass exams.

- You will not be asked questions in an exam on material that you have not discussed in class. Exams are not there to trick you, but for you to demonstrate an understanding of the subject.
- Revise! Revise! Revise!
- Plan your time so that your revision is done in small chunks; usually an hour per night is enough, so that you are focused on what you are revising, remain motivated and do not lose sight of your goal of passing the exam first time.
- Make use of the notes you have made in class and in your independent study time.
- Revise in a group and pick one topic to revise each week before the exam.
- Practise timed exam questions at home.
- Attend mock exams if these are held or complete online exams that may be an optional part of your module work.

The day before

- Don't try to revise at all.
- Check the time of the exam and where it is being held.
- If you are using public transport, check the times of the bus or train; if your other commitments allow, plan to get an earlier bus or train than you would normally.
- Check you have all the equipment necessary for the exam, for example pencils, pens, erasers, your student ID card and a bottle of water.
- Try to relax, and get an early night so that you awake refreshed in the morning. Avoid caffeine and large amounts of alcohol the night before, as this will only prevent you sleeping and may cause you to feel groggy in the morning.

As an active learner you will find that exams and assignments will still pose a challenge to you, but the above advice is about learning to deal with them in a way that enables you to enjoy your course and develop an understanding of the under-pinning theories as they apply to practice.

Assessment of practice

Practice is assessed throughout your course and you will have to meet the require-ments of the NMC as a fit and competent practitioner at the point of registration. This point is important as many of the criticisms of nurse education after nursing became a university-based course were that students were not fit for practice at the end of three years and could not carry out basic care for patients. You may remember the 'too posh to wash' debate last year, when this criticism was again raised in the media. The Peach Report (UKCC, 1999) identified this as a problem when evaluating students who had graduated from nursing courses after the introduction of Project 2000. There have been many changes to practice assessments over the past five years, but the following conditions currently apply.

- All students will have mentor and possibly a co-mentor who will supervise them in practice and with whom they will work for at least 15 hours per week.
- Students will have supernumerary status – this means that they will not be part of the rostered number of staff on duty.
- All students need to have experience of 24-hour care – this means that students will need to work the shifts with their mentor or co-mentor to gain that experience. This includes night duty and working at weekends.
- Students will have to keep a portfolio of their experience to show to their mentor and to their personal tutor.
- The NMC (2007b) requires students to have an Ongoing Achievement of Practice Record, which will go with you from placement to placement. This is shared with your mentors and will include comments from them. The final mentor that you will have is known as the 'sign-off' mentor and he or she will be responsible for signing off to say that you have met the competences for registration.

Mentors

Mentors are nurses who have undergone further education to take on this role. You will recall from earlier in this chapter that we discussed the *NMC Code of Professional Conduct*; if you revisit standard 6.4, you will see that all registered nurses have a duty to facilitate students' learning and achievement of competence. Thus any registered nurse you will work alongside will do their best to help you gain confidence and competence.

Mentors have other responsibilities for you and your fellow students.

- They will help you construct a learning contract that can be tailored to meet your needs and to meet the competences you have to achieve.
- They can help you gain other learning opportunities while working in their areas of practice. For example, you may work with other health professionals, such as occupational therapists, in the care of clients.
- They will make a judgement about your performance and assess your practice against the competences you have to achieve. Mentors will talk to other members of the clinical team with whom you have worked to gain a rounded picture of your performance.

- They will give you feedback on your performance, both in a positive light and to offer areas for improvement in your performance for your next placement.
- They also have a responsibility, if you are not meeting the expected standards of performance, to work with individuals who support learners in practice and with your personal tutor to help you achieve these. You will not always gain competence in practice at the first attempt, but there are many ways in which you can be helped and many people willing to help you.

Being an active learner in placements is just as important as it is at university; this involves applying the characteristics of active learning to a clinical placement. Be enthusiastic and read around the type of clients or patients you may expect to meet in the area you are going to. Meet your mentor before you start your placement; that first introduction is important as it demonstrates enthusiasm, interest and commitment to your mentor. The relationship you have with your mentor is pivotal in ensuring that you are able to meet your competences and make the most of your placement. Mentors are passionate about the clients and patients they work with and will expect students to show the same respect and empathy as they do.

Mentors all have a sense of responsibility for their students, so are concerned if students exhibit the following behaviours:

- lack of enthusiasm;
- turning up late for shifts or being unable to work shifts because of other commitments;
- not attempting to make contact with the clinical area before beginning a placement;
- making disparaging remarks about the clients or patients.

If you reflect on this negative approach to placement learning, you can see why you may not get as much from the placement as other students who demonstrate more active learning styles. Enter with a positive attitude, willing to learn and willing to work with your mentor. This will facilitate your learning in practice, your clinical skills development and your enjoyment and success in practice.

Portfolios

The main purpose of a portfolio is for you to be able to demonstrate your application of the theory you have learnt to a practice setting. When you are qualified, your portfolio acts as a way of recording your nursing career and professional development and is a requirement of the NMC for all registered nurses. Portfolios are another way to demonstrate how becoming an active learner aids you in developing competence and skills in practice, and in becoming a lifelong learner. Nairn et al. (2006) undertook a study to consider how student nurses used portfolios and found that they helped students by offering them ways to develop their own learning, reflection and coping strategies, and found them a useful part of career development. Both Nairn et al. and Scholes et al. (2004) also looked at the drawbacks in using portfolios; for example, students were not always sure what should be included in them, and they were not always reviewed by their mentors and personal tutors so potential learning opportunities and the opportunity to help students link theory to practice were missed.

Despite these well-founded criticisms, portfolios are an important way to demonstrate learning.

Activity 8.8

*   Think about what types of evidence of learning you will need to put in your portfolio; be as creative as you like.
*   Write down a list of the evidence.
*   Also write down what might not be helpful to include in a portfolio, although this may be a by-product of your learning experience.

There is a brief outline answer at the end of the chapter.

A framework can be offered to help you start this part of your learning, but use it as a way to show how you have managed to achieve your learning outcomes. To this end, portfolios should include:

*   a brief résumé of your career to date;
*   an analysis of your strengths and areas for development;
*   evidence of your achievement of a cross-branch experience;
*   evidence of your achievement of each practice competency for registration and progression from the CFP to your branch programmes;
*   learning contracts;
*   reflections;
*   records of tutorials and records of achievement at the end of each year;
*   skills development profiles.

Things that are less helpful include: copies of your assignments, although feedback is helpful in demonstrating you have taken account of it and have developed or addressed the issues in future work; and leaflets from placements or areas you have visited – although useful to you they do not demonstrate achievement.

You will need to be able to discriminate as to what you put in and leave out of your portfolio. This is the type of discussion that can be had with your personal tutor and your mentor in placements, as they are able to offer you help and advice on this.

Ongoing Achievement of Practice Record

The Ongoing Achievement of Practice Record is a new requirement from the NMC and will be given to you along with your portfolio and assessment of practice competence. The suggestions by the NMC for the use of this document fit in with the way most practice assessment is carried out with your mentor. Following are some of the key points and the roles and responsibilities of mentors, students and the university as described by the NMC (2007b).

- The student and mentor meet together at the end of a placement to document strengths, development needs and any concerns. The document is to be shared with the education provider.
- The student is to be responsible for carrying the documentation from placement to placement with copies retained by the education provider.
- Within five days of commencing a placement, the documentation is to be used by the student and mentor to formulate a developmental plan and set goals that take account of strengths, issues and concerns raised in previous placements.
- Regular meetings are scheduled to evaluate progress by student and mentor throughout a placement (involving academic staff when appropriate), at least at the midpoint and at the end of a placement, where strengths and any issues for development are addressed.
- Where a specific development plan has been put in place and concerns remain, then an evaluation session with the mentor must be scheduled urgently and others involved as appropriate, e.g. academic staff.
- Where there are causes for concern, a student representative might also be present.

As you can see, these are the roles and responsibilities of the mentor, with the addition of the sharing of this record and their comments with your personal tutor and the mentor on your next placement.

Stress

Starting a university nursing course and meeting new people on practice placements can both cause stress, which is a physiological and psychological response to stressors. For example, you may feel very stressed by the thought of an exam or being assessed in practice. While this is a natural reaction to some events, it becomes problematic when individuals are not able to use effective coping mechanisms to deal with it (Kozier et al., 2008). Stress affects people emotionally, psychologically, physically and socially, from feeling anxious about everyday events to affecting your relationships with your friends and family. People deal with stress differently, by using various coping mechanisms. You can see from this chapter that becoming an active learner can help you reduce the stress you may encounter during your course. The strategies used to increase your learning are at the same time good coping mechanisms for dealing with the stress of the course. An example could be taking an exam: an effective revision pattern will enable you to feel confident in being able to take the exam successfully; however, cramming creates stress and anxiety because you are not sure if you will know enough information to pass.

Many students may experience financial hardship while on the programme and this can be a source of considerable stress and anxiety for them. While part of being a student is learning to manage your own budget, universities are very aware that this is a potential problem for students. All universities do offer support services from debt counselling to hardship funds which students can apply to for financial help. It is important to recognise that this is an issue with which universities have a great deal of expertise and these services are there to help and support you.

Universities want their students to succeed and there are times when life events and circumstances may affect how well a student performs in their academic and clinical work. Your programme will recognise that such events do occur and all universities put in provisions to help students in such cases. These are known as extenuating circumstances and all universities will have procedures which will allow you to submit these and not be penalised for events beyond your control. As ever, your personal tutor is your first port of call.

The student handbook is an invaluable and often overlooked resource which contains all the vital information for submitting extenuating circumstances to the penalties attached to academic misconduct, i.e. plagiarism. Students often file this away on day one and never revisit the contents until something dreadful happens, but it is worth reading through the contents as this will enable you to be aware of the support available should you encounter difficulties during the programme.

It is important to recognise in yourself when you are becoming stressed and whether this is having a detrimental effect on your life; for example, feeling overwhelmed by work, becoming anxious over everyday events such as catching a bus, avoiding friends or not taking part in normal social activities. There are many sources of help and advice, from family and friends, to your personal tutor or your GP, and all universities have professional counselling services available to help you.

Kozier et al. (2008) suggest some of the following strategies to help you cope:

- daily planned relaxation;
- a regular exercise routine;
- learning to accept failure, yours and others';
- forming a support network of friends and colleagues;
- talking about the things that are causing you stress with someone you trust and who can understand.

Psychological well-being is equally as important as physical health when undertaking nursing courses and it is important you look after yours, and to recognise it in your colleagues and others on your course.

CHAPTER SUMMARY

- Entering nursing as a university student is a life-changing experience and you need to prepare yourself and your significant others before you undertake this step. This can be by a thorough exploration of your chosen pathway and by considering the impact that this will have on you emotionally and physically.
- Nursing is a profession that has an emerging knowledge base, and it is regulated by a code of standards and ethics in caring for patients' clients and their families.
- Becoming an active learner in both theoretical components and the practice experience will enable you to be successful, reduce your stress and plan time effectively, so that you can enjoy your life.

Activities: brief outline answers

8.2 Nursing knowledge (page 152)

If we take as an example a patient who is admitted with a chest infection:

- epistome may be the use of drugs to control infection: types, dosages and side effects;
- technes may include drug administration, or making the patient comfortable;
- phronesis may include experience of the patient and their ability to take medications, and what to do if the patient refuses medication.

8.4 Code of Professional Conduct (page 155)

You may have looked at several examples of the *Code* here:

- Treating people as individuals.
- Ensuring you gain consent.
- Working with others to protect and promote the health and well-being of those in your care, their families and carers and the wider community.

These are three elements of the *Code*; however, all standards refer to the care of patients, clients and their families. You can see that the *Code* and the implications for practice as a registered nurse permeate every aspect of the care and interaction you have with all patients, carers and their families, and that it is a key guide to the expectations of the behaviour and performance of a registered nurse.

8.7 Essay title analysis (page 163)

The aspects you should have thought about include:

- how many words are required;
- what the title means by communication, for example verbal or non-verbal;
- what else needs to be included; for example, if you are going to nurse children, the communication would be different from that you would use with a person who has a mental health problem or an adult with a learning disability;
- what 'discuss' means as opposed to 'describe';
- what you already know about the subject;
- whether communication is the most important aspect of care and, if so, why.

8.8 Portfolios (page 168)

Portfolios are individual to the person; as each person's experience is different their portfolios will not be the same, and this is how it should be. However, this makes it scary as there is no set formula and no one way to get it right, unlike a lot of other aspects of nursing. As an active learner you can take control of your portfolio and think how to construct it so that it reflects you as an individual and how you have achieved the outcomes in practice.

Knowledge review

Having completed the chapter, how would you now rate your knowledge of the following topics?

	Good	Adequate	Poor
1. How I can become an active learner			
2. The implications of professional regulation for registered nurses			
3. How I can make the most of the learning opportunities in practice			
4. How I can ensure that I know how to manage my work–life balance			

Further reading

Clay, G (2003) Assignment writing skills. *Nursing Standard* 17(20): 47–52, 54–5.

Crow, J (2005) Preparing your assignment – referencing your work. *Practice Nurse* 30(1): 41–3.

Davison, N (2005) Writing good essays: a life-long skill. *Nursing Times* 101(4): 62–3.

Maslin-Protheroe, S (2005) *Study Skills for Nurses and Midwives*, 3rd edition. Edinburgh: Balliere Tindall.

Useful websites

www.bbc.co.uk/keyskills This website has many useful tips on learning styles and a learning styles questionnaire which is quick and easy to complete.

www.brainbox.co.uk This is an excellent site which offers a variety of material on learning styles and a modified Honey and Mumford questionnaire. It is free to use and has many valuable learning and teaching resources, including a good maths page.

www.nmc.uk The official website of the Nursing and Midwifery Council – the governing body for nurses and midwives.

www.rcn.org.uk Royal College of Nursing website.

www.vark-learn.uk Details of the VARK (visual, aural, read/write and kinesthetic) learning style.

Chapter 9

Conclusions and future directions

Future policy and organisational directions

In preceding chapters we have seen how NHS policy and organisation have developed over the years. Several developments are on the horizon at the time of writing, which are likely to have an impact on nurses and their careers as we progress through the early twenty-first century. These are briefly summarised below and there are links suggested to appropriate websites for further reading.

The reconfiguration of hospital services

It seems likely that there will be some further reorganisation of all NHS services but what form this will take is still unknown. Many NHS organisations are consulting and their plans may mean ward and service closures and relocations. It is possible that the centralisation of acute services, such as A & E departments, may take place in big 'supercentres'; and that chronic care and diagnostic services may be undertaken in non-hospital settings and closer to patients' homes. The King's Fund (2006) outlines the drivers for these change as:

- the pressure to achieve financial balance across the NHS;
- the introduction of the government's recent policy to move more care out of hospitals and into the community in order to improve efficiency and access;
- the reorganisation of care on the grounds of evidence that some services are safer when delivered in certain configurations;
- the need to respond to external changes, such as the extension of the European Working Time Directive to cover the hours of junior doctors.

Opinion has it that the government agenda will ultimately move the NHS from a state-owned organisation that both purchases and provides services, to one where there is a large number of autonomous public and private organisations within a tightly regulated healthcare market so that a wide range of institutions exert influence on the quality of care. As the Labour government has pushed these types of reforms further than its predecessors, it is likely that this trend will continue, with the expansion of Foundation Trusts, independent treatment centres and a growing role for the independent sector, aimed at improving patient choice. However, the extent to which the NHS and, more specifically, its staff can tolerate further change is debatable (Lewis et al., 2006).

Our NHS, our future

Lord Darzi, a prominent surgeon and Parliamentary Undersecretary of State for Health, was asked to the review progress of the Labour government's reforms and concluded (Darzi, 2007) that, as of 2007, the NHS was two-thirds of the way through the reform programme set out since 2000; that people generally had little enthusiasm for radical change such as, for example, a health service based on private insurance rather than taxation; but that improving the quality of service delivery would take further fundamental change and local accountability. The NHS has already, Darzi argues, improved considerably as a result of record investment levels, even if patients, staff and the public do not always recognise this. The NHS will become:

- fair and available to all, but could do more to reduce health inequalities and so further NHS action is outlined to achieve this;
- personal, with greater regard to patient choice within the system; plans are outlined to expand GP and health centre services with more flexible provision, including evening and weekend opening hours;
- effective, giving patients outcomes that are top quality; the Health Innovations Council is recommended to promote innovation;
- safe, to give the public confidence in NHS services; further work needs to be done in incident reporting, inspecting hospitals, increasing the powers of Matrons, and introducing MRSA screening.

A second stage of the review will set out how this vision for the NHS can be achieved across eight areas:

- maternity and newborn care;
- children's health;
- planned care;
- mental health;
- staying healthy;
- long-term conditions (LTCs);
- acute care;
- end-of-life care.

Darzi (2007) also believes that the NHS would benefit from a greater distance from the political process, and recommends that an NHS Constitution should be drawn up to achieve this.

Practice-based commissioning

Practice-based commissioning (PBC) is an idea that has been around for nearly ten years but has yet to be fully implemented. It is the devolution of commissioning (buying services) away from PCTs to general practice teams who would have accountability for how the money is spent as well as budgets (Lewis et al., 2007). The idea is to secure:

- a greater variety of services;
- services delivered by a greater number of providers and in settings that are closer to home and more convenient to patients;
- more efficient use of services;
- greater involvement of front-line doctors and nurses in commissioning decisions;
- a strengthening of the power of commissioners relative to the providers; that is, increasing GP practice teams' power in relation to the hospitals with whom they contract.

PBC is intended to place better emphasis on prevention and health promotion rather than cure (Lewis et al., 2007), and is likely to have some impact on the location and provision of services in the future.

Modernising nursing careers

Christine Beasley (DH, 2006d), the Chief Nursing Officer for England, outlines directions in which nurses and the nursing profession should move as healthcare demands change in line with social changes. These contextual changes include:

- a more complex society with greater diversity;
- larger numbers of people living to greater ages;
- lifestyle issues, such as obesity and lack of exercise, that contribute to morbidity and mortality;
- the continuation of health inequalities;
- a smaller working population in relation to their dependents;
- higher expectations of health services among the population;
- rapid advances in treatments that are costly;
- review and reform of services, with greater patient choice, individual care pathways and more emphasis on health promotion.

She argues that, as society changes, so nursing and the way in which nurses work will have to change. Nurses will continue to care for those who cannot care for themselves, for whatever reason, and to promote health, and the key elements of practice, education, quality and leadership will always remain, but in the future nurses will need to respond to social change by:

- organising care around patients' needs;
- ensuring that good-quality nursing care is delivered, with high productivity and value for money;
- working across hospital and community care, using telemedicine and working in organisations other than the NHS, with advanced skill levels;
- being skilled enough to care for older people and those with LTCs;
- being able to use health promotion;
- working in and leading multidisciplinary teams;
- working with those in new roles, such as assistant practitioners.

In order to do this, the priorities will be to develop a competent and flexible work-force, update career pathways, prepare nurses to lead, and modernise the public image of nursing.

The future nurse

The RCN (2004) has also outlined its vision for the future of nursing, in which the challenges for nursing are spelled out in a similar tone to those of *Modernising Nursing Careers* (DH, 2006d). They see the purpose of nursing as being to provide holistic healthcare for patients, families, carers and communities; and being responsible for improving health, facilitating recovery and, where appropriate, ensuring a dignified death. For the RCN, nursing has a particular:

- **purpose**: promoting health and preventing disease, illness, injury and disability;
- **mode of intervention**: empowering people;
- **knowledge domain**: people's experiences of health-related events;
- **focus**: on the whole person;
- **value base**: expressed in a code of ethics and professional regulation;
- **commitment to partnership**: with patients, carers, communities and with other team members.

The RCN sees its role as leading nursing into the future, in three action areas: first, by recognising nursing as a family including unqualified members of staff and carers; second, with a focus on person-centred care as a central philosophy; and, third, by working across care settings. In order to achieve this, they call for nurses with a high level of skills and graduate entry as the requirement for registration, and they seek to achieve this through influencing public life and political debate.

Nursing: towards 2015

The NMC commissioned Longley et al. (2007) to examine possible future scenarios for nursing and nurse education, and their literature review discusses healthcare and health policy issues, and their impact on nursing and nurse education. Many of the concepts relating to social change have already been discussed in this book but, specifically regarding nurse education, they argue that recruitment and retention are still pressing issues, and the 'four branches' structure (with distinct programmes for adult, child health, mental health and learning disabilities nursing) is questioned, with a future education structure based around specialism a possibility. They contrast the service needs for a more generic worker (with broader skills crossing today's professional boundaries) with the need for specialisation. All-graduate entry is argued to be a way forward to enhance the status of nursing in relation to other professions, with greater inter-professional education a priority.

They outline three scenarios for the future nursing workforce, with the extent of qualified nurses' specialisation a central issue.

- **'Steady as she goes'**: with a small number of specialist nurses in relation to other qualified staff and healthcare assistants, as is the case currently.
- **'More specialisms for all'**: with a greater number of specialist nurses and fewer other qualified staff and a similar number of healthcare assistants compared to currently, with other specialist roles taken by non-nurses.
- **'No more generalists'**: where all qualified nurses are specialists, supported by advanced healthcare assistants and a similar number of healthcare assistants as currently.

These scenarios were put out for consultation in November 2007.

Quality assurance

A new process for quality assurance and enhancement of practice settings and higher education institutions (HEIs) is due to be introduced in 2008. This is called EQUIP (Enhancing Quality in Partnership). It is being led by Skills for Health, the UK government agency responsible for equipping health sector workers with skills to support service development and delivery (see www.skillsforhealth.co.uk). The proposals (Skills for Health, 2007) should have a major impact on quality assurance and development in placement learning, and is a big issue on the horizon for those working for NHS Trusts, the private sector and HEIs. Government and professional bodies' policies have emphasised the importance of clinical experience for HCPs, including nurses (DH, 1999b, 2001c; QAA, 2001). Latterly, there has been a focus on how this can be quality assured across multiple professions, how the review processes can be streamlined and simplified (QAA, 2003), and how effective action can be taken at local level to make sure that improvements come about (DH, 2005b; Williamson et al., 2008). HEIs and practice placement providers will share a framework of standards for monitoring and programme review, including learning taking place in both campus and practice-based settings. In order to achieve this, user-friendly and achievable standards called 'requirements' have been developed after an extensive national consultation process, against which quality will be measured for the management and delivery of healthcare education programmes. This will clarify the organisations' responsibilities and raise the profile of placement learning, making it easier for placement providers to document, share and improve their student support activities, according to one pilot study (Williamson et al., 2008). The requirements have a broad emphasis (Skills for Health, 2007) under seven headings.

- Values.
- Evaluating, maintaining and improving quality.
- Resources, management and governance.
- Teaching and learning.
- Student selection, progression and achievement.
- Student/learner support.
- Assessment.

Quality in healthcare: future considerations

The delivery of high-quality care and treatment should be at the very heart of all healthcare provision in both the NHS and the independent sector. Judgements about what constitutes good quality of care centre largely on the experience of holistic care, which meets the needs of individuals by treating them and respecting them as people and by involving them in decision-making processes. Government reforms have aimed to tackle wider issues, such as inequalities in health and the improvement of service provision across a wide range of conditions, including cancer. The report entitled *The State of Health Care* (Healthcare Commission, 2007) indicates that, while many improvements have been made, particularly in the reduction of waiting times and the incidence of HAIs, much still needs to be done to create a service that is world class. In particular, there remains concern over how to reduce the inequalities in health that certain groups experience. The findings of this report will act as further incentives to improve practice in the next decade or so.

While it goes without saying that quality assurance is ongoing across the NHS, surely future considerations must be given to the care of older people. Thanks largely to improvements in standards of living and important advances in medicine and various surgical interventions during the latter half of the twentieth century, most of us can now expect to live into old age. However, with increased longevity comes the possibility of a greater incidence of chronic illness. There is a concern that, although we may be living longer, more of us are living with LTCs such as asthma, arthritis and diabetes. The over 65s are currently the NHS's biggest client group and are continuing to increase in number, yet standards of care for this cohort are at best variable. Growing concerns over the quality of care have the led to the implementation of an NSF for Older People and the introduction of EOC benchmarks to improve practices with this client group. Specific aspects of care, such as nutrition for older people and respect for their privacy and dignity at vulnerable times, are at the forefront of the agenda for change. This must remain a key focus for decades to come as more generations pass through this life stage. This is an ongoing challenge for healthcare workers from all professions in the NHS.

In conjunction with raising actual physical standards of care delivery, there is also a need to raise individual performance standards. This involves examining one's own personal values, beliefs and attitudes about nursing the elderly, as, for so long, elderly care has been of little consequence in the overall provision of care in the NHS. The eradication of ageist practices in healthcare that discriminate against people because of their age is outlined in Standard One of the NSF and typifies the commitment within healthcare to improve the older person's experience of the service. The recommendations of the Healthcare Commission's report, *Caring for Dignity* (2007), have considerable implications for the future nursing of older people. For far too long these important aspects have been overlooked and the poor quality of service provision simply accepted. The quality of people who work with the sick elderly also needs to improve so that, where possible, enthusiastic, motivated and knowledgeable clinicians, who are seen to engage in a meaningful way with older people, are involved in their care. There is a need for clinicians who are respectful of clients, who value them as individuals, who acknowledge their autonomy to make decisions and who encourage them to participate in care activities. Education has an important part to play in raising standards, by informing and enthusing nurses with knowledge of developments in practice and the need to remain up to date with current thinking and develop strategies for challenging poor practice performance.

The introduction of the Modern Matron role has begun to address some of these issues through strong leadership, leading by example and encouraging others to follow. Through reminding and encouraging nurses to raise standards, it is hoped that older people will receive the type of care that causes them no harm. Good leaders are needed in all aspects of nursing older people – leaders who can inspire, engender confidence and transform practice. Attitudes towards working with older people among some sections of the healthcare workforce have in the past been rather negative and work with this client group has been seen as hard and unrewarding. This unfortunate view has to led to many practitioners not wanting to work with older people, leaving those who do often under-resourced and pressured. Sometimes people with inappropriate attitudes find work with this client group and, in certain circumstances, this can lead to abuse of the vulnerable older person. These are people who misunderstand their role as caregivers, have little interest in their client group and may view ageing and the aged very negatively – poor-quality people delivering poor-quality care. These attitudes must change as we embrace an era of an unprecedented increase in human longevity in which most people can expect to live into their seventies and beyond. If the quality of care for this client group is to improve, then attitudes, often deep-seated ageist attitudes, must be challenged and replaced by a much more optimistic and humanitarian approach to care delivery and treatment. Therein, perhaps, lies the greatest challenge of all in the decades to come – the challenge of each and every one of us to change our views about ageing and the aged, otherwise we too will succumb to the negativity that has so beset the generations before us.

The patient perspective: future considerations

The expectations of people who use the health service are changing. More emphasis is now placed on choice and patient satisfaction than ever before. Patients with LTCs are even encouraged to become experts, advising and teaching others about the best ways to cope with and manage their conditions. No longer are doctors and nurses seen as the sole providers of expert knowledge, for the relationship between the patient and professional has changed to one of a partnership, involving people in their own care and treatment, and helping them make choices and decisions.

Listening to the patient perspective has become an integral part of this new relationship. This has involved not only a change in role but also a change in attitude towards patients, away from the old 'doing to' dependent model of healthcare, to one of participation and self-care management. The future decades will continue to see a rise in this type of relationship in order to continue effecting better control over conditions that, in the main, cost the NHS millions of pounds to treat every year. Central to these reforms is a belief in the respect for autonomy, that is, the power of the individual to make decisions about circumstances that affect them personally. This will include a gradual recognition of the rights of the individual to discuss their wishes regarding end-of-life decisions and will see increased use of living wills or advanced directives to guide actions at this time of life.

Patients have a unique perspective on the quality of care provision. They will continue to be consulted regarding the care experience and their views will be used to shape and improve service provision for the future. Important insights into how people wish to be treated and cared for by healthcare staff are gleaned through patient satisfaction surveys and by consulting with patient groups. The dialogue is ongoing and evolving in the pursuit of quality in care. Professionals will need to continue listening to the patient's perspective so as to tailor healthcare interventions that meet the patient's needs. Paternalism no longer has a place in healthcare, although some patients will still prefer that the doctor or nurse takes over, with a 'you know best nurse', whenever they are asked to participate in care decisions. While there is nothing wrong with this if it is the patient's way of coping with difficult situations, generally people expect much more involvement and to be consulted about their care in the twenty-first century. The government's commitment to modernising the NHS since the late 1990s has the patient perspective at the heart of its reforms. The old-fashioned ways of working in the NHS are changing, hierarchies are being flattened and patients are having more say and are more involved in their own care. It yet remains to be seen if this will result in overall greater satisfaction, reduced costs and complications, and better self-care management for the future, but the sentiment is a noble one nonetheless.

Useful websites

www.kingsfund.org.uk The King's Fund is an independent charity that conducts health-related research.
www.nmc-uk.org Nursing and Midwifery Council website.
www.ournhs.nhs.uk Up-to-date information about the progress of Our NHS, Our Future.
www.skillsforhealth.org.uk/page/quality-assurance Skills for Health quality assurance pages.

References

Abel-Smith, B (1960) *A History of the Nursing Profession*. London: Heinemann.

Acheson, D (1998) *Independent Inquiry into Inequalities in Health Report*. London: Stationery Office.

Adams, J (1994) Opportunity 2000. *Nursing Times*, 20 April (90): 16.

Anionwu, E (2006) *About Mary Seacole*. Available online at www.maryseacole.com/maryseacole/pages/aboutmary.html (accessed 28 March 2007).

Atkinson, FI (2000) Survey design and sampling, in Cormack, D (ed.) *The Research Process in Nursing*. Oxford: Blackwell Science.

Attree, M (2001) Patients' and relatives' experiences and perspectives of 'good' and 'not so good' quality care. *Journal of Advanced Nursing*, 33(4): 456–66.

Baggott, R (2004) *Health and Health Care in Britain*, 3rd edition. Basingstoke: Palgrave Macmillan.

Baggott, R (2007) *Understanding Health Policy*. Bristol: The Policy Press.

Ball, J (2006) *Nurse Practitioners 2006*. London: Royal College of Nursing.

Basford, L (1995) Module 1: Focus of care, in Basford, L and Slevin, O, *Theory and Practice of Nursing: An integrated approach to patient care*. Edinburgh: Campion Press.

Bassett, C (2002) Nurses' perceptions of care and caring. *International Journal of Nursing Practice*, 8(1): 8–15.

Benner, P (1984) *From Novice to Expert: Excellence and power in clinical nursing practice*. Menlo Park, CA: Addison-Wesley.

Benner, P and Wrubel, J (1989) *The Primacy of Caring: Stress and coping in health and illness*. Wokingham: Addison-Wesley.

Beveridge, W (1942) *Social Insurance and Allied Services Report*. Presented to Parliament by command of His Majesty. London: HMSO.

Blakemore, K (1998) *Social Policy: An introduction*. Buckingham: Open University Press.

Bolton, SC (2000) Who cares? Offering emotion work as a gift in the nursing labour process. *Journal of Advanced Nursing*, 32(3): 58–66.

Boult, C and Allen, D (1997) Last minute election promises on health. *Nursing Standard*, 11(32): 7.

Bradley, H (1994) Gendered jobs and social inequality, in *The Polity Reader in Gender Studies*. Oxford: Polity Press.

Broussard, BB (2005) Women's experiences of bulimia nervosa. *Journal of Advanced Nursing*, 49(1): 43–50.

Buchan, J and Seccombe, I (2004) *Fragile Future? A review of the UK nursing labour market in 2003.* London: Royal College of Nursing.

Bulmer, M, Lewis, J and Piachaud, D (1989) *The Goals of Social Policy.* London: Unwin Hyman.

Burns, T and Sinfield, S (2003) *Essential Study Skills: The complete guide to success at university.* London: Sage.

Bury, T and Mead, J (1998) *Evidence-based Health Care: A practical guide for therapists.* Oxford: Butterworth-Heinemann.

Butler, RN (1975) *Why Survive? Growing old in the United States.* New York: Harper and Row.

Caelli, K, Ray, L and Mill, J (2003) 'Clear as mud': toward greater clarity in generic qualitative research. *International Journal of Qualitative Methods*, 2(2). Article 1. Available online at www.ualberta.ca/~iiqm/backissues/pdf/caellietal.pdf (accessed 4 July 2007).

Cancer Research UK (2008) *Breast Cancer Key Facts* webpages. Available online at http://info.cancerresearchuk.org/cancerstats/types/breast/ (accessed 18 March 2008).

Carlisle, C, Kirk, S and Luker, KA (1996) The changes in the role of the nurse teacher following the formation of links with higher education. *Journal of Advanced Nursing*, 24: 762–70.

Carnwell, R (2000) Essential differences between research and evidence-based practice. *Nurse Researcher*, 8(2): 55–68.

Carper, BA (1978) Fundamental patterns of knowing. *Nursing Advances in Nursing Science*, 1(1): 13–23.

Carruthers, I (2006) *Strengthening Commissioning. Gateway 6569.* London: Department of Health.

Carter, DA (2000) Quantitative research, in Cormack, DFS (ed.) *The Research Process in Nursing*, 4th edition. Oxford: Blackwell Science.

Carter, DA and Porter, S (2000) Validity and reliability, in Cormack, DFS (ed.) *The Research Process in Nursing*, 4th edition. Oxford: Blackwell Science.

Carveth, JA (1995) Perceived patient deviance and avoidance by nurses: what should nurses do to reduce difficulties? *Nursing Research*, 44: 173–7.

Chapman, CM (1998) Is there a correlation between change and progress in nursing education? *Journal of Advanced Nursing*, 28(3): 459–60.

Clinical Governance Support Team (2008) *About Clinical Governance* web pages. Available online at www.cgsupport.nhs.uk/ (accessed 16 March 2008).

Commission for Healthcare Audit and Inspection (CHAI) (2005) *Inspecting, Informing, Improving: About the Healthcare Commission.* London: CHAI.

Commission for Healthcare Audit and Inspection (CHAI) (2007) *Caring for Dignity: A national report on dignity in care for older people in hospital.* London: CHAI.

Cooke, M, Chaboyer, W, Schluter, P and Hiratos, M (2005) The effect of music on preoperative anxiety in day surgery. *Journal of Advanced Nursing*, 52(1): 47–55.

Corby, S (1995) Opportunity 2000 in the National Health Service, *Employee Relations*, 17(2): 23–37.

Cormack, D (2006) *The Research Process in Nursing*, 5th edition. Oxford: Blackwell Science.

Cottrell, S (2008) *The Study Skills Handbook*. Basingstoke: Palgrave Macmillan.

Critical Appraisal Skills Programme (CASP) and the Health Care Libraries Unit (1999) *Evidence Based Health Care Workbook*. Oxford: Update Software.

Cronin, P, Rawlings-Anderson, K (2004) *Knowledge for Contemporary Nursing Practice*. Edinburgh: Mosby.

Cutcliffe, JR and McKenna, HP (1999) Establishing the credibility of qualitative research findings: the plot thickens. *Journal of Advanced Nursing*, 30(2): 374–80.

Darzi, A (2007) *Our NHS, Our Future*. Interim report, Department of Health. Available online at www.dh.gov.uk/en/Publicationsandstatistics/Publications/Publications PolicyAndGuidance/dh_079077 (accessed 27 November 2007).

Davies, C (1995) *Gender and the Professional Predicament in Nursing*. Buckingham: Open University Press.

Department of Health (DH) (1989) *Working for Patients. Working Paper 10: Education and training*. London: HMSO.

Department of Health (DH) (1992) *The Patients' Charter*. London: Department of Health.

Department of Health (DH) (1997) *The New NHS – Modern, Dependable*. London: HMSO.

Department of Health (DH) (1998a) New NHS for patients takes shape – family doctors and community nurses put in the driving seat. Press release 98/262. Available online at www.coi.gov.uk/coi/depts/GDH (accessed 2 November 1998).

Department of Health (DH) (1998b) *A First Class Service: Quality in the new NHS*. London: HMSO.

Department of Health (DH) (1998c) *The Health of the Nation: A policy assessed*. London: Department of Health. Available online at www.publications.doh.gov.uk/pub/docs/doh/exec/pdf (accessed 14 September 2007).

Department of Health (DH) (1999a) *Saving Lives: Our healthier nation*. Available online at www.archive.official-documents.co.uk/document/cm43/4386/4386.htm (accessed 14 February 2007).

Department of Health (DH) (1999b) *Making a Difference: Strengthening the nursing, midwifery and HV contribution to health and health care*. London: HMSO.

Department of Health (DH) (1999c) New opportunities for NHS Direct. Press release 99/227. Available online at www.coi.gov.uk/coi/depts/GDH/coi4144f.ok (accessed 2 November 1999).

Department of Health (DH) (1999d) *Clinical Governance in the New NHS*. London: HMSO.

Department of Health (DH) (2000) *The NHS Plan: A plan for investment, a plan for reform*. London: HMSO. Available online at www.dh.gov.uk (accessed 14 February 2007).

Department of Health (DH) (2001a) *National Service Framework for Older People*. London: HMSO.

Department of Health (DH) (2001b) *The Essence of Care: Patient focused benchmarking for healthcare professionals*. London: HMSO.

Department of Health (DH) (2001c) *Placements in Focus: Guidance for education in practice for healthcare professions*. London: ENB.

Department of Health (DH) (2001d) *The Expert Patient: A new approach to chronic disease management for the 21st century.* Norwich: Stationery Office.

Department of Health (2002) *Developing Key Roles for Nurses and Midwives: A guide for managers.* London: Department of Health.

Department of Health (DH) (2003a) *Modern Matrons: Improving the patient experience.* London: Department of Health.

Department of Health (DH) (2003b) *Tackling Health Inequalities: A programme for action.* Available online at www.dh.gov.uk/en/Publicationsandstatistics/ Publications/PublicationsPolicyAndGuidance/DH_4008268 (accessed 21 September 2007).

Department of Health (DH) (2004) *NHS Improvement Plan: Putting people at the heart of public services.* Norwich: Stationery Office.

Department of Health (DH) (2005a) *National Service Framework for Long Term (Neurological) Conditions.* Norwich: Stationery Office.

Department of Health (DH) (2005b) *Ongoing Quality Monitoring and Enhancement Guidance.* Available online at www.dh.gov.uk (accessed 24 May 2004).

Department of Health (DH) (2006a) *Health Reform in England: Update and next steps.* London: Department of Health.

Department of Health (DH) (2006b) *Primary Care Trust and Stategic Health Authority Roles and Functions. Gateway 6566.* Available online at www.dh.gov. uk/en/Publicationsandstatistics/Publications/PublicationsPolicyAndGuidance/ DH_4134649 (accessed 4 July 2007).

Department of Health (DH) (2006c) *The Health Act,* chapter 28. Available online at www.opsi.gov.uk/ACTS/acts2006/20060028.htm (accessed 20 March 2007).

Department of Health (DH) (2006d) *Modernising Nursing Careers: Setting the direction.* London: Department of Health.

Department of Health (DH) (2006e) *Learning from Bristol: The Department of Health's response to the Report of the Public Inquiry into children's heart surgery at the Bristol Royal Infirmary 1984–1995.* London: HMSO. Available online at www.dh.gov.uk/en/Publicationsandstatistics/Publications/PublicationsPolicy AndGuidance/Browsable/DH_4111999 (accessed 15 October 2007).

Department of Health (DH) (2006f) *Dignity in Care,* Practice Guide 09. London: Social
· Care Institute for Excellence.

Department of Health (DH) (2007a) *Foundation Trusts.* Available online at www.dh. gov.uk/PolicyAndGuidance/OrganisationPolicy/SecondaryCare/NHSFoundation Trust/fs/en (accessed 12 February 2007).

Department of Health (DH) (2007b) *Primary Care* web pages. Available online at www.dh.gov.uk/en/Aboutus/HowDHworks/DH_074639 (accessed 4 July 2007).

Department of Health (DH) (2007c) Reid 'green lights' £4 billion investment for new hospitals. Press release. Available online at www.dh.gov.uk/en/Publicationsand statistics/Pressreleases/DH_4086620 (accessed 21 September 2007).

Department of Health (DH) (2007d) Progress of new hospital schemes approved to go ahead. Available online at www.dh.gov.uk/en/Procurementandproposals/Public privatepartnership/Privatefinanceinitiative/index.htm (accessed 21 September 2007).

Department of Health (DH) (2007e) *Agenda for Change* web pages. Available online at www.dh.gov.uk/en/Policyandguidance/Humanresourcesandtraining/Modernising pay/Agendaforchange/index.htm (accessed 20 March 2007).

de Wit, R and van Dam, F (2001) From hospital to home care: a randomized controlled trial of a Pain Education Programme for cancer patients with chronic pain. *Journal of Advanced Nursing*, 36(6): 742–54.

Donnan, PT (2000) Experimental research, in Cormack, D (ed.) *The Research Process in Nursing*. Oxford: Blackwell Science.

Douglas, F, van Teijlingen, E, Torrance, N, Fearn, P, Kerr, A and Meloni, S (2006) Promoting physical activity in primary care settings: health visitors' and practice nurses' views and experiences. *Journal of Advanced Nursing*, 55(2): 159–68.

Edwards, N (2005) Can quality improvement be used to change the wider health care system? *Quality and Safety in Health Care*, 14(2): 75.

Egan, G (1998) *The Skilled Helper: A problem management approach to helping*, 6th edition. Pacific Grove, CA: Brooks Cole.

Eraut, M (1994) *Developing Professional Knowledge and Competence*. London: Routledge Falmer.

EU Parliament and Council (2005) *Recognition of Professional Qualifications*, Directive 2005/36/EC, 7 September. EU Parliament and Council: Brussels

Florence Nightingale Museum Trust (2003) *Florence Nightingale*. Available online at www.florence-nightingale.co.uk/flo2.htm (accessed 28 March 2007).

Ford, P and Walsh, M (1995) *New Rituals for Old: Nursing through the looking glass*. Oxford: Butterworth-Heinemann.

Francis, B and Humphreys, J (1998) The commissioning of nurse education by consortia in England: a quasi-market analysis. *Journal of Advanced Nursing*, 28(3): 517–23.

Freidman, M and Friedman, R (1980) *Free to Choose*. London: Penguin.

Garrett, L and Clarke, A (2008) *Get Ready for A & P for Nursing and Health Care*. Harlow: Pearson Education.

Gibbs, G (1998) *Learning by Doing: A guide to teaching and learning methods*. London: Further Education Unit.

Goffman, E (1961) *Asylums*. London: Pelican.

Gray, R, Rofail, D, Allen, J and Newey, T (2005) A survey of patient satisfaction with and subjective experiences of treatment with antipsychotic medication. *Journal of Advanced Nursing*, 52(1): 31–7.

Griffin, M and Melby, V (2006) Developing an advanced Nurse Practitioner service in emergency care: attitudes of nurses and doctors. *Journal of Advanced Nursing*, 56(3): 292–301.

Griffiths, R (1983) *NHS Management Inquiry: Report to the Secretary of State of Social Services*. London: HMSO.

Gustavsson, B (2004) Revisiting the philosophical roots of practice knowledge in editors, in Higgs, J, Richardson, B and Abrandt-Dahlgren, M (eds) *Developing Practice Knowledge for Health Professionals*. Edinburgh: Butterworth-Heinemann.

Hall, C (2006) Curb on Alzheimer's Drugs. *The Daily Telegraph*, 26 February 2006. Available online at www.telegraph.co.uk/news/main.jhtm?xml=/news/2006/05/27/nalz27.xml (accessed 11 October 2007).

Halligan, L (2007a) Ten years of going round in circles. *The Sunday Telegraph.* Available online at www.telegraph.co.uk/news/main.jhtml?xml=/news/2007/02/25/nrhewitt125.xml (accessed 24 April 2008).

Halligan, L (2007b) Half of hospitals delay surgery to save cash. *The Sunday Telegraph.* Available online at www.telegraph.co.uk/news/main.jhtml?xml=/news/2007/02/25/nhs25.xml (accessed 24 April 2008).

Harrison, S, Hunter, DJ, Marnoch, G and Pollitt, C (1992) *Just Managing: Power and culture in the NHS.* Basingstoke: Macmillan.

Hayek, FA (1960) *The Constitution of Liberty.* London: Routledge and Kegan Paul.

Healthcare Commission (2007) *The State of Health Care.* London: Healthcare Commission.

Healthcare Commission (2008) About us: what is the Healthcare Commission and why do we exist? Available online at www.healthcarecommission.org.uk (accessed 16 March 2008).

Hek, G and Moule, P (2006) *Making Sense of Research: An introduction for health and social care practitioners.* London: Sage.

Hicks, N (1997) Evidence-based health care. *Bandolier,* 4(39): 8.

Higher Education Funding Council for England (HEFC) (2001) *Strategies for Widening Participation in Higher Education: A guide to good practice.* London: HEFC.

HM Treasury (2007) *Public Private Partnerships: The private finance initiative.* Available online at www.hm-treasury.gov.uk (accessed 21 September 2007).

Hochschild, AR (2003) *The Managed Heart: Commercialization of human feeling.* Twentieth Anniversary edition. Berkeley, CA: University of California Press.

Holliday, ME and Parker, DL (1997) Florence Nightingale, feminism and nursing. *Journal of Advanced Nursing,* 26: 483–8.

Hunter, B (2001) Emotion work in midwifery: a review of current knowledge. *Journal of Advanced Nursing,* 34(4): 436–44.

Hutchings, A, Williamson, GR and Humphreys, A (2005) Supporting learners in clinical practice: capacity issues. *Journal of Clinical Nursing,* 14(8): 945–55.

Hutton, W (1996) *The State We're In.* London: Vintage.

Hyde, V, Jenkinson, T, Koch, T and Webb, C (1999) Constipation and laxative use in older community dwelling adults. *Clinical Effectiveness in Nursing,* 3(4): 170–80.

Illiffe, S and Munro, J (eds) (1997) *Healthy Choices: Future options for the NHS.* London: Lawrence and Wishart.

International Council of Nurses (ICN) (2006) *The ICN Code of Ethics for Nurses.* Available online at www.icn.ch/icncode.pdf (accessed 15 October 2006).

Jenkinson, T (1996) Surgical nursing: the nurse as significant other for surgical patients. *Professional Nurse,* 11(10): 651–2.

Johnson, A (2007) BBC Breakfast News, 18 September 2007.

Johnson, M (2003) Ethnic diversity in health and social context, in Kai, J (ed.) *Ethnicity, Health and Primary Care.* Oxford: Oxford University Press.

Johnson, M and Webb, C (1995) Rediscovering unpopular patients: the concept of social judgement. *Journal of Advanced Nursing,* 21(3): 466–75.

Kai, J (ed.) (2003) *Ethnicity, Health and Primary Care.* Oxford: Oxford University Press.

Kai, J and Bhopal, R (2003) Ethnic diversity in health and disease, in Kai, J (ed.) *Ethnicity, Health and Primary Care.* Oxford: Oxford University Press.

Kelly, M and May, D (1982) Good and bad patients: a review of the literature and theoretical critique. *Journal of Advanced Nursing*, 7: 147–56.

Kennedy, I (2001) *The Inquiry into the Management of Care of Children Receiving Complex Heart Surgery at the Bristol Royal Infirmary.* Bristol: Bristol Royal Infirmary. Available online at www.bristol-inquiry.org.uk (accessed 15 October 2007).

King's Fund (2006) *The Reconfiguration of Hospital Services.* Available online at www.kingsfund.org.uk/publications/briefings/the_1.html (accessed 27 November 2007).

Klein, R (2006) *The New Politics of the NHS*, 5th edition. London: Longman.

Kozier, B, Erb, G, Berman, A, Snyder, S, Lake, R and Harvey, S (2008) *Fundamentals of Nursing Concepts, Process and Practice.* Harlow: Pearson Education.

Kyle, TV (1995) The concept of caring: a review of the literature. *Journal of Advanced Nursing*, 21: 506–14.

Lambert, V (2007) Why the NHS will never add up. *The Daily Telegraph.* Available online at www.telegraph.co.uk/health/main.jhtml?xml=/health/2007/02/26/hnhs26.xml (accessed 13 March 2007).

Leathard, A (2000) *Health Care Provision Past, Present and Into the 21st Century*, 2nd edition. Cheltenham: Stanley Thornes.

Lewis, R, Alvarez-Rosete, A and Mays, N (2006) *King's Fund.* Available online at www.kingsfund.org.uk/publications/kings_fund_publications/how_to_regulate.html (accessed 27 November 2007).

Lewis, R, Curry, N and Dixon, M (2007) *Practice-based Commissioning: From good idea to effective practice.* King's Fund. Available online at www.kingsfund.org.uk/publications/kings_fund_publications/practicebased.html (accessed 27 November 2007).

Lincoln, YS and Guba, EG (1984) *Naturalistic Inquiry.* Newbury Park, CA: Sage.

Liu, JE, Mok, E and Wong, T (2006) Caring in nursing: investigating the meaning of caring from the perspective of cancer patients in Beijing, China. *Journal of Advanced Nursing*,15(2): 188–96.

Longley, M, Shaw, C and Dolan, G with Stackhouse, R (2007) *Nursing: Towards 2015. Alternative scenarios for healthcare, nursing and nurse education in the UK in 2015.* Available online at www.nmc-uk.org/aArticle.aspx?ArticleID=2641 (accessed 4 December 2007).

Long Term Conditions Alliance (LTCA) (2006/7) Time to take stock. *Connect*, 32(Winter).

Macdonald, M (2007) Nurse–patient encounters: constructing harmony and difficulty. *Advanced Emergency Nursing Journal*, 29(1): 73–81.

Magne, P. (2004) *Learning Development Student Pack.* University of Plymouth, NHSU, Dorset and Somerset SHA, South West Peninsula SHA.

Marshall, TH and Bottomore, TB (1992) *Citizenship and Social Class.* London: Pluto Press.

Marsland, D (1996) *Welfare or Welfare State?* Basingstoke: Macmillan.

McCartney, J (2006) A terrible country in which to grow old. *The Daily Telegraph*, 15 October 2006. Available online at www.telegraph.co.uk/opinion/main.jhtml?xml=/opinion/2006/10/15/do1507.xml (accessed 11 October 2007).

McCaughan, E and McKenna, H (2007) Never-ending making sense: towards a substantive theory of the information-seeking behaviour of newly diagnosed cancer patients. *Journal of Clinical Nursing* (OnlineEarly Articles). Available online at doi:10.1111/j.1365–2702.2006.01817.x.

McGauran, A (2002) News extra: parliamentary committee criticizes PFI. *British Medical Journal*, 325: 124.

McPherson, W, Cook, T, Setamu, J and Stone, R (1999) The Inquiry into matters arising from the death of Stephen Lawrence. Available online at www.archive.official-documents.co.uk/document/cm42/4262/sli-pre.htm (accessed 29 April 2008).

McSherry, R and Haddock, J (1999) Evidence-based health care: its place within clinical governance. *British Journal of Nursing*, 8(2): 113–17.

McVicar, A (2003) Workplace stress in nursing: a literature review. *Journal of Advanced Nursing*, 44(6): 633–42.

Means, R and Lart, R (1994) User empowerment, older people and the UK reform of community care, in Smith, R and Raistrick, J (eds) *Policy and Change*. Bristol: School of Advanced Urban Studies.

Mill, JS (2001) *Utilitarianism*, 2nd edition. Indianopolis, IN: Hackett Publishing.

Ministry of Health and Scottish Home and Health Departments (1966) *Report of the Committee on Senior Nursing Staff Structure (the Salmon Report)*. London: HMSO.

Monti, EJ and Tingen, MS (1999) Multiple paradigms of nursing science. *Advances in Nursing Science*, 21(4): 64–80.

Moore, A (1998) Clinical equals. *Nursing Standard*, 12(27): 24–5.

Moore, D (2005) *Assuring Fitness for Practice: A policy review commissioned by the Nursing and Midwifery Council Nursing Task and Finish Group*. London: NMC.

Mulcahy, L (2003) *Disputing Doctors: The socio-dynamics of complaints about medical care*. Buckingham: Open University Press.

Nairn, S, O'Brien, E, Traynor, V, Williams, G, Chapple, M and Johnson, S (2006) Student nurses' knowledge, skills and attitudes towards the use of portfolios in a school of nursing. *Journal of Clinical Nursing*, 15: 1509–20.

National Statistics Population Trends (2006) 126 (Winter). Available online at www.statistics.gov.uk/ (accessed 20 April 2007).

NHS and Community Care Act (1990). London: HMSO. Available online at www.opsi.gov.uk/ACTS/acts1990/Ukpga_19900019_en_1.htm (accessed 26 June 2007).

NHS Employers (2007) *Gender Equality Duty*. Available online at www.nhsemployers.org/excellence/excellence-403.cfm (accessed 18 April 2007).

NHS Executive (NHSE) (1996) *Promoting Clinical Effectiveness: A framework for action in and through the NHS*. London: Department of Health.

NHS Executive (NHSE) (1998a) *Information on Clinical Effectiveness*. London: NHSE.

NHS Executive (NHSE) (1998b) *Clinical Effectiveness Resource Pack*. London: NHSE.

NHS Executive (NHSE) (1998c) *Working Together: Securing a quality workforce for the NHS*. London: HMSO.

NHS Executive (NHSE) (1999a) *Clinical Governance in the New NHS*. London: NHSE.

NHS Executive (NHSE) (1999b) *Making a Difference: Strengthening the nursing, midwifery and health visiting contribution to health and healthcare*. Available online at www.dh.gov.uk/en/Publicationsandstatistics/Publications/Publications PolicyAndGuidance/DH_4007977 (accessed 20 July 2007).

NICE (2005) *A Guide to NICE*. London: National Institute for Health and Clinical Excellence.

NICE (2007) *Technology Appraisal 111: Alzheimer's disease – donepezil, galantamine, rivastigmine (review) and memantine: guidance (amended September 2007)*. London: National Institute for Health and Clinical Excellence.

Northouse, PG (1979) Interpersonal trust and empathy in nurse–nurse relationships. *Nursing Research*, 28(6): 365–7.

Nurses, Midwives and Health Visitors Act (1979) Chapter 24. London: HMSO.

Nursing and Midwifery Council (NMC) (2002a) *Guidelines for Records and Record Keeping*. London: NMC.

Nursing and Midwifery Council (NMC) (2002b) *Supporting Nurses and Midwives Through Lifelong Learning*. London: NMC.

Nursing and Midwifery Council (2004) *Standards of Proficiency for Pre-registration Nursing Education*, London: NMC.

Nursing and Midwifery Council (NMC) (2006a) *Standards to Support Learning and Assessment in Practice*. London: NMC.

Nursing and Midwifery Council (NMC) (2006b) *Revision to NMC Circular 37/2005, Pre-registration Nursing Programmes: Progression for the Common Foundation Programme (CFP) to Branch*. NMC circular 16/2006. London: NMC.

Nursing and Midwifery Council (NMC) (2007a) *Introduction to Essential Skills Clusters for Pre-registration Nursing Programmes*. NMC circular 07/2007. Available online at www.nmc-uk.org/circulars (accessed 16 March 2008).

Nursing and Midwifery Council (NMC) (2007b) *Ensuring Continuity of Practice Assessment Through the Ongoing Achievement Record*. NMC Circular 33/20. Available online at www.nmc-uk.org/circulars (accessed 16 March 2008).

Nursing and Midwifery Council (2008) *The NMC Code of Professional Conduct: Standards for conduct, performance and ethics*. London: NMC. Available online at www.nmc-uk.org (accessed 16 March 2008).

Oakley, A (1981) *Subject Women*. Oxford: Martin Robertson.

Paley, J (2001) An archaeology of caring knowledge. *Journal of Advanced Nursing*, 36(2), 188–98.

Papadopoulos, I (ed.) (2006) *Transcultural Health and Social Care: Development of culturally competent practitioners*. Oxford: Elsevier.

Parahoo, K (2006) *Nursing Research Principles, Processes and Issues*, 2nd edition. Basingstoke: Palgrave Macmillan.

Parsons, T (1951) *The Social System*. London: Routledge and Kegan Paul.

Parsons, T (1956) *Family, Socialization and Interaction Process*. London: Routledge and Kegan Paul (with Robert Bales).

Patel, S (2003) Mental health, in Kai, J (ed.) *Ethnicity, Health and Primary Care*. Oxford: Oxford University Press.

Phillips, S (1996) Labouring the emotions: expanding the remit of nursing work? *Journal of Advanced Nursing*, 24(1): 139–43.

Plastow, L, Luthra, M, Powell, R, Wright, J, Russell, D and Marshall, MN (2001) Head lice infestation: bug busting vs. traditional treatment. *Journal of Clinical Nursing*, 10(6): 775–83.

Porter, S (1992) Women in a women's job: the gendered experience of nurses. *Sociology of Health and Illness*, 14(4): 510–27.

Porter, S (2000) Qualitative research, in Cormack, DFS (ed.) *The Research Process in Nursing*, 4th edition. Oxford: Blackwell Science.

Pyne, RH (1998) *Professional Discipline in Nursing, Midwifery and Health Visiting*, 3rd edition. Oxford: Blackwell Science.

Quality Assurance Agency (QAA) (2001) *Code of Practice for the Assurance of Academic Quality and Standards in Higher Education: Placement learning*. London: QAA.

Quality Assurance Agency (QAA) (2003) *Streamlining Quality Assurance in Healthcare Education*. Available online at www.qaa.ac.uk (accessed 24 May 2005).

Quinn, FM (1995) *The Principles and Practice of Nurse Education*, 3rd edition. Cheltenham: Stanley Thornes.

Rafferty, AM (1996) *The Politics of Nursing Knowledge*. London, Routledge.

Richardson, B, Higgs, J and Abrandt-Dahlgren, M (2004) Recognising practice epistemology in the health professions, in Higgs, J, Richardson, B and Abrandt-Dahlgren, M (eds) *Developing Practice Knowledge for Health Professionals*. Edinburgh: Butterworth-Heinemann.

Rivett, GC (1998) *From Cradle to Grave: Fifty years of the NHS*, online edition. London: King's Fund. Available online at www.nhshistory.net/index.html (accessed 8 February 2007).

Rivett, GC (2007) *National Health Service History: Nursing.* Available online at www.nhshistory.net/nursing.htm#Nursing (accessed 3 October 2007).

Rosenthal, R and Jacobson, L (1968) *Pygmalion in the Classroom: Teacher expectation and pupils' intellectual development*. New York: Holt, Rinehart and Winston.

Rowntree, D (1988) *How to Study: A guide for students of all ages*. London: Warner Books.

Royal College of Nursing (RCN) (2004) *The Future Nurse: The RCN vision*. London: RCN.

Royal College of Nursing (RCN) (2005a) *NHS Knowledge and Skills Framework Outlines for nursing posts*. Available online at www.rcn.org.uk/publications/pdf/ NHS%20knowledge%20and%20skills%20framework/pdf (accessed 20 March 2007).

Royal College of Nursing (RCN) (2005b) *Nurse Practitioners.* Available online at www.nursepractitioner.org.uk/Documents/NursePractitioners.pdf (accessed 16 February 2007).

Russell, WH (1857) Preface, in Seacole, M, *Wonderful Adventures of Mrs Seacole in Many Lands.* London: James Blackwood. Available online at http://digital.library. upenn.edu/women/seacole/adventures/adventures.html#VIII (accessed 28 March 2007).

Sackett, DL, Rosenberg, WMC, Gray, JAM, Haynes, RB and Richardson, WS (1996) Evidence-based medicine: what it is and what it isn't. *British Medical Journal*, 312: 71–2.

Sackett, DL, Strauss, SE, Richardson, WS, Rosenberg, WMC and Haynes, RB (1997) *Evidence Based Medicine: How to practise and teach EBM*. Cheltenham: Churchill Livingstone.

Sandford, D (2003) *Why Bristol Is So Important*. BBC News. Available online at http://news.bbc.co.uk/1/hi/health/1443081.stm (accessed 15 October 2007).

Scally, G and Donaldson, LJ (1998) Clinical governance and the drive for quality improvement in the new NHS in England. *British Medical Journal*, 317: 61–5.

Scholes, J, Webb, C, Gray, M, Endicott, R, Miller, C, Jasper, M and McMullan, K (2004) Making portfolios work in practice. *Journal of Advanced Nursing*, 46(6): 595–603.

Seedhouse, D (1994) *Fortress NHS: A philosophical review of the NHS*. London: Wiley and Sons.

Sheaff, M (2005) *Sociology and Health Care: An introduction for nurses, midwives and allied health professionals*. Buckingham: Open University Press.

Skills for Health (2007) EQUIP: *Enhancing quality in partnership: healthcare education QA consultation framework*. Available online at www.skillsfor health.org.uk/uploads/page/364/uploadablefile.pdf (accessed 20 November 2007).

Staden, H (1998) Alertness to the needs of others: a study of the emotional labour of caring. *Journal of Advanced Nursing*, 27(1): 147–56.

Stein, L (1967) The doctor–nurse game. *Archives of General Psychology*, 16: 699–703.

Stein, L, Watts, D, and Howell, T (1990) The doctor–nurse game revisited. *New England Journal of Medicine*, 322(8): 546–9.

Steven, A (1999) Named nursing: in whose best interest? *Journal of Advanced Nursing*, 29(2): 341–7.

Stockwell, F (1972) *The Unpopular Patient*, The Study of Nursing Care: Series 1. London: RCN.

Stuart, A (undated) *Mary Seacole: The real angel of the Crimea*. Available online at www.channel4.com/culture/microsites/O/origination/who_was_mary_seacole.ht ml (accessed 28 March 2007).

Tilki, M (2006) Human rights and health inequalities: UK and EU policies and initia-tives relating to the promotion of culturally competent care, in Papadopoulos, I (ed.) *Transcultural Health and Social Care: Development of culturally competent practitioners*. Oxford: Elsevier.

Timmons, S and Tanner, J (2005) Operating theatre nurses: emotional labour and the hostess role. *International Journal of Nursing Practice*, 11(2): 85–91.

Titmuss, RM (1976) *Commitment to Welfare*. London: Allen and Unwin.

Townsend, P, Davidson, N and Whitehead, M (1992) *Inequalities in Health: The Black Report and the health divide*. London: Penguin Books.

Toynbee, P (2007) NHS: the Blair years. *British Medical Journal*, 334: 1030–1. Available online at http://bmj.com/cgi/content/full/334/7602/1030 (accessed 22 May 2007.

United Kingdom Central Council for Nursing, Midwifery and Health Visiting (UKCC) (1999) *Fitness for Practice: The UKCC Commission for Nursing and Midwifery Education*, London: UKCC.

van Hooft, S (2006) *Caring About Health*. Aldershot: Ashgate Publishing.

Wall, A and Owen, B (2002) *Health Policy*, 2nd edition. London: Routledge.

Walsh, M and Ford, P (1992) *Nursing Rituals, Research and Rational Actions*. Oxford: Butterworth-Heinemann.

Walsh, M and Walsh, A (1999) Measuring patient satisfaction with nursing care: experience of using the Newcastle Satisfaction with Nursing Scale. *Journal of Advanced Nursing*, 29(2): 307–15.

Wanless, D (2002) *Securing our Future Health: Taking a long-term view*. London: HM Treasury. Available online at www.hm-treasury.gov.uk/wanless (accessed 21 September 2007).

Wanless, D, Appleby, J, Harrison, A and Patel, D (2007) *Our Future Health Secured? A review of NHS funding and performance*. Available online at www.kingsfund. org.uk/publications/kings_fund_publications/our_future.html (accessed 18 September 2007).

Watson, J (2002) *Assessing Caring in Nursing and Health Science*. New York: Springer Publishing.

Watson, J (2006) Can an ethic of caring be maintained? *Journal of Advanced Nursing*, 54(3): 257–9.

Webb, C and Hope, K (1995) What kind of nurse do patients want? *Journal of Clinical Nursing*, 4(2): 101–8.

Webster, C (2002) *The National Health Service: A political history*, 2nd edition. Oxford: Oxford University Press.

White, R (1976) Some political influences surrounding the Nurses Registration Act 1919 in the United Kingdom. *Journal of Advanced Nursing*, 1: 209–17.

Williams, C (2007) Unpopular patients in the intensive care unit: is holistic care achievable? *Nursing in Critical Care*, 12(2): 59–60.

Williamson, GR (2004) Illustrating triangulation in nursing research. *Nurse Researcher*, 12(4): 7–18.

Williamson, GR, Webb, C and Abelson-Mitchell, N (2004) Developing lecturer practitioner roles using action research. *Journal of Advanced Nursing*, 47(2): 153–64.

Williamson, GR, Collinson, S and Withers N (2007) Patient satisfaction audit of a nurse-led lung cancer follow-up clinic. *Cancer Nursing Practice*, 6(8): 31–5.

Williamson, GR, Heath, V, Ballantyne, E, Callaghan, L, Webster, D and Hunter, C (2008) Improving student support in professional placement learning: lessons from the South West Peninsula Pilot of a new national placement evaluation process. *The Open Nursing Journal*, 2: 21–7.

Work and Families Act (2006) Chapter 18. London: HMSO.

Index